GET ON THE BALL
FOR GREAT ABS

GET ON THE BALL FOR GREAT ABS: *Exercises to Flatten Your Stomach and Strengthen Your Core*

Copyright © 2006 by Lisa Westlake

Published by Marlowe & Company
An Imprint of Avalon Publishing Group, Inc.
245 West 17th Street, 11th Floor
New York, NY 10011

A V A L O N
publishing group incorporated

First published as *Strong and Stable* by
ABC Books in Australia in 2007. This edition
published by arrangement.

Library of Congress Cataloging-in-Publication
Data is available from the publisher.

ISBN-13: 978-1-56924-260-5
ISBN-10: 1-56924-260-7

9 8 7 6 5 4 3 2 1

Printed in Singapore

GET ON THE BALL
FOR GREAT ABS

Exercises to Flatten Your Stomach and Strengthen Your Core

Lisa Westlake

Marlowe & Company
New York

CONTENTS

GET RESULTS,
GET MOVING, GET FIT

Are you looking for an exercise program that gives your abdominals and core muscles an exceptional workout? A workout that will simultaneously shape the rest of your body from top to bottom, that can be done anywhere, anytime, and delivers fabulous results?

Get on the Ball for Great Abs will help you use an exercise ball to strengthen and define visible muscles, especially your abs, for a great-looking body while also focusing on the muscles that are essential for devoloping your body's core control. Core control is the ability of specific deep muscles to support the spine, shoulders and pelvis. Strengthening your core helps keep your back healthy and provides you with the foundations required to tone and strengthen your abdominals, plus arms, thighs, butt, and more. Enjoy the feeling of well-being as you become fitter, stronger and more flexible.

Get on the Ball for Great Abs builds on the basic ball techniques introduced in *Get on the Ball* to provide a new range of ball exercises suitable for all ages and fitness levels. Whether you have already discovered the benefits of ball workouts and are looking for more, or you are just discovering this innovative training tool, *Get on the Ball for Great Abs* will provide you with options to suit your goals and ability.

So you want fab abs

Whether you want a toned, taut torso or you're looking to improve your back health there is a major focus on abdominals in almost every exercise in *Get on the Ball for Great Abs*.

There are four layers of abdominals. The outer layers, rectus abdominis and the external and internal obliques are important for strength and definition. The deepest layer, the transversus abdominis, may be invisible, but it plays a major role, with other deep muscles, in the stability and integrity of the spine. Poor function of these muscles is closely related to back pain and injury. To simplify the approach to ab training, think of these layers as the outer movers and the inner stabilizers. So which should you train?

Refine and boost your fitness program

Once upon a time, we all thought that crunches and sit-ups were the key to abdominal tone and the ever-elusive six-pack. Today we know there is a better way. Working out on an exercise ball will help you not only look great and feel fantastic; it will give you a stronger, leaner, injury-free body.

Strength alone does not make the man or woman

With the knowledge that sensible exercise plays a role in the prevention of illness and injury, a comprehensive approach to fitness has been developed in *Get on the Ball for Great Abs* embracing the value of core stability, balance, joint mobility and flexibility.

Training core abdominals is for everyone.

Everyone's back is vulnerable. Including deep abdominal strengthening in your workout helps to protect your back and provides underlying stability that allows you to take your training further. A major bonus of ball training is the inclusion of deep abdominal activatement in almost every exercise. If you have a weak or injured back core stability should be your focus, as outer ab curls and crunches may exacerbate your problem.

Should you aim for "six-pack abs"?

If your goal is a "lean machine, washboard look," and your back is healthy, you'll love the ab curls, crunches and hovers in the abdominal section of *Get on the Ball for Great Abs*. The ball provides added challenge and variety to traditional ab curls. You'll feel the difference!

To see those rippling abs, low body fat is required. While you can hone in on strengthening an area to lose body fat around your midsection, you must lose it everywhere. This is why a mixed exercise program will still help you achieve your goals.

SO WHAT
IS NEW?

Great ways to keep you strong, stable and able

While exercising on a ball has been used for rehabilitation for over 40 years, its fitness applications have evolved over the past decade. An exercise ball is a great way to add variety and challenge to your workouts. *Get on the Ball for Great Abs* introduces new exercise techniques and programs on the ball, specifically designed to strengthen your core, develop your abdominals and improve overall body tone and fitness.

More than 80 new exercises

Get on the Ball for Great Abs will show you a range of ways to safely and effectively use the exercise ball to optimize your fitness, stability and balance. *Get on the Ball for Great Abs* offers variations and progressions to the basic ball exercises, such as those in *Get on the Ball*.

Upbeat warm-up and cardio choices

Low impact cardio and warm-up options are also included in your ball training repertoire. Gentle mobility warm-ups are for everyone. If you like to get your heart rate going and have a little fun on the ball, you'll love the energy as you bounce into action.

Bands and balls

Using lightweight resistance bands is an inventive, convenient and effective way to perform strength conditioning on the ball. Easy to follow band and ball exercises provide fantastic strength and muscle definition and are the perfect alternative to using hand weights, to mix up your training program.

Focus on posture, balance and control

The magic of the exercise ball workout is that it gives you more than muscle tone. Important elements of health and fitness are enhanced by ball exercises. These exercises will provide you with new ways to improve your balance, core stability, back health and posture.

Custom-designed training programs

Create your own training session or select from the pre-designed workouts to suit your needs. Whether your goal is to strengthen your abdominals, tone your upper arms, firm that butt, focus on stretching or gentle exercise, or care for your weak back or working out post-pregnancy, there's a program for you. Take a look at the new innovative 10-minute "quick-fix" programs especially for a morning wake-up, an evening cool down or to combat common problems caused by working long hours at a computer.

BALL
BENEFITS

Why work out on a stability ball?

Using an exercise ball provides a range of improved alternatives to exercising on terra firma. Training on an unstable base "wakes up" muscles you don't normally use, facilitating strength, balance and core stability providing a healthy toned body, inside and out. Responding to the fluidity of the ball also helps your muscles gain mobility and flexibility to keep your body supple and moving with ease.

Get on the Ball for Great Abs provides a broad scope of exercises that enhance:

> Flexibility for freedom of movement.

> Strength for function, form and a great looking physique.

> Core stability providing you with a healthy back and strong foundations for healthy, injury-free movements in every day physical and athletic activities.

> Cardiovascular health boosting the performance of your heart and lungs.

> Balance, decreasing the risk of trips and falls, helping you perform with improved ability and control.

> Posture as the ball encourages muscle control and a finer focus on exercise.

SOMETHING
FOR EVERYONE

One person's warm-up is another person's workout

Whether you're a gym junkie, exercise ball pro, or you're new to the concept of ball fitness, *Get on the Ball for Great Abs* has a range of options to suit your individual needs.

You may like to ease into your session with gentle mobility on the ball, or you may prefer to bounce into action with a more upbeat warm-up. Each exercise features an option to increase or decrease load and instability for all levels of training. Build your own workout or select one of maximum fitness programs to suit your specific goals and abilities.

Listen to your body and choose what's right for you.

Take care

Get on the Ball for Great Abs is designed *to help* people of all ages and levels of fitness. However, it is not a rehabilitation manual.

> If you are injured or have a medical condition you may need extra guidance in designing the right exercise program for your needs and limitations.

> If you are using ball exercises to assist a condition be sure to discuss appropriate exercise selection with your healthcare provider.

> If you have a new illness or injury you must seek professional assessment and treatment before commencing or continuing any exercise.

HEALTH
AND FITNESS

It takes total-body fitness to get great abs

A comprehensive fitness program today includes more than a dash of cardio exercise and lifting a few weights. Postural awareness, core stability, balance, mobility and flexibility are also important additions to the total fitness portfolio. Attention to good form, breathing and relaxation are also important. Finally, we must not forget the most key ingredients in the recipe for exceptional health and fitness: nutrition, hydration, rest and relaxation, variety, commitment, and motivation.

Put it all together and you get an energized mind and a body and mind that looks and feels fantastic. Let's take a look at the total health and fitness recipe.

Nutrition

Fuel your fitness regime with a healthy diet composed of plenty of fresh vegetables and fruit, nutritious whole grains and sensible servings of lean proteins such as fish, chicken and occasional red meat.

Hydration

Be sure to drink 6 to 8 glasses of water a day to stay hydrated.

Rest and relaxation

Lack of sleep leaves you less likely to maintain healthy eating and exercise patterns and makes you more inclined to let your fitness program laps. Pleny of R&R will make help you stay focused on healthy habits.

Variety

Varying your daily training and weekly workout will help you beat boredom and avoid overstressing any particular body part. When you approach your exercise program, your body and mind need to be kept motivated. Try different ball exercises and programs and compliment these with other activities such as cycling, swimming, yoga or Pilates.

Commitment
This is the best gift you can give to yourself. It's your life and you deserve good health, vitality and to feel terrific. Invest in your future, put your body first and make the time to exercise.

Motivation
Fitness doesn't happen overnight but the more you do, the more incentive you will have to keep you working toward your goals. A few helpful hints to keep you going include:

> Making and revising short-term targets, such as "each day I will do extra repetitions in my exercise program," may be more effective than concentrating on one huge goal, such as "I want a six-pack by the end of the month."

> Be realistic and patient. The motto "good things come to those who wait" is particularly true of exercise programs.

> Create a list of reasons why you want to be fit, strong and feel fabulous. Put this list on your fridge or office wall as a reminder of your goals.

> Find a friend. Band together to commit to a workout time and long term exercise plan.

Remember a fit, healthy body takes effort but the outcome is invaluable.

WHAT THE BALL
CAN DO FOR YOU

Fitness for your heart and lungs

Cardiovascular exercise improves the function of your heart, lungs and circulation. It helps to boost your metabolism, which is essential for maintaining your optimum body weight.

Get on the Ball for Great Abs includes low impact cardiovascular exercise options that can be used as a workout or warm-up. These exercises will get you ready for your exercise ball strengthening work and will also help to raise your fitness levels. You may like to include other cardiovascular exercise such as walking, running, swimming, cycling, rollerblading or rowing. Just 20 to 30 minutes a day, 3 to 5 times a week will improve your fitness. Start out gently then gradually add a little extra speed or distance as your endurance improves.

Balanced strength for perfect posture

Strength conditioning is beneficial for maintaining healthy bones, controlling your weight and enhances your ability to perform general activities without strain or injury. Working muscles against resistance gives you a stronger, toned body and taller posture — so you will look good too.

It is important to balance your strength training program by working all muscles equally. Avoid the "mirror muscle syndrome" that is the temptation to focus on anterior (front) muscles just because they are stronger and more visible. Giving equal respect and dedication to the weaker posterior (back) muscles will give you a stronger core region and help avoid muscle imbalances that can lead to slouching and injury.

Move it or lose it

Mobility and flexibility is your best form of health insurance. Joint stiffness and tight muscles restrict your body's quality of movement and can lead to injuries. Use the gentle mobility exercise ball options to warm-up and cool down. Sprinkle them among your strength exercises on the ball to keep your joints supple and to maintain a full range of body movement.

Add a stretching routine to your weekly exercise program. This will help to improve your flexibility, but more importantly prevent injury to ligaments and tendons by improving muscular elasticity. Always stretch every muscle worked in an exercise session. You will find stretches to accompany each ball exercise or you can do them at the end of a training session.

Stretch at the end of exercise, and your body will thank you for many, many years to come.

STABILITY
AND BALANCE

Stability

The ability of deep muscles to switch on to stabilize the spine, shoulder blades, hips and pelvis is essential for safe, effective exercise. Strong core control improves the body's ability to bear the brunt of activities that might otherwise cause pain or injury.

The exercise ball is an ideal way to unite core stability with regular training. Just like a house, no matter how grand and beautiful the outside looks, without strong foundations, it will collapse.

Stabilizing muscles in the abdominal region are vital for healthy movement. The reason why these muscles are often neglected as they cannot be seen and are often hard to feel. Take a look at "Engaging the Core" on page 26 to help you find and use these muscles correctly.

Balance

Our ability to avoid falling when we slip or trip, respond quickly to the spin on a tennis ball, and to perform every day life and sporting activities with ease and confidence all rely on great balance. Our reaction time can start to decline in our thirties and beyond so it makes sense to inject a little balance training into regular workouts.

The exercises in *Get on the Ball for Great Abs* all work to improve balance and movement awareness.

Get on the ball for a body that stands tall, moves gracefully and is strong both inside and out.

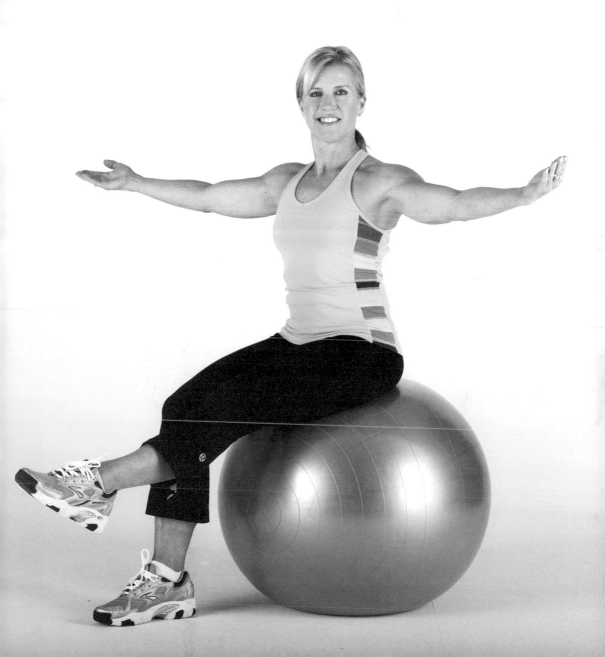

HOW MANY, HOW HEAVY, HOW OFTEN

Weights, bands and repetitions

Load and number of repetitions are provided with each exercise as a guide only. You will know you have the right combination when you can feel your muscle working hard, but you are able to complete that last rep with fine form. Be sure to maintain excellent technique. If you feel discomfort other than muscles working or your form is compromised you need to decrease the load, instability or number of reps.

Use the following table as a guide to how heavy your weights should be. Bands are color-coded according to their resistance level but every brand is different. If you are fit and healthy, you are likely to benefit from a medium band, but if you are new to exercise or not so strong, start out with the lighter band and follow the "listen to your body" principle as you progress.

EXPERIENCE	LEVEL 1	LEVEL 2	LEVEL 3
BACK, NECK OR SHOULDER PAIN INJURED, PREGNANT	NO WEIGHTS	NO WEIGHTS	NO WEIGHTS
STARTING OUT ON THE BALL NO WEIGHT TRAINING EXPERIENCE	NO WEIGHTS	NO WEIGHTS	2.5 LB/1 KG
MINIMAL EXPERIENCE ON BALL OR WITH WEIGHTS	NO WEIGHTS	2.5 LB/1 KG	5 LB/2 KG
COMFORTABLE WITH BASIC BALL EXERCISES OR WORKED A LITTLE WITH WEIGHTS	2.5 LB/1 KG	5 LB/2 KG	7 LB/3 KG
CONFIDENT ON THE BALL AND WORKED WITH WEIGHTS	5 LB/2 KG	7 LB/3 KG	10 LB/4 KG
OFTEN WORKS WITH WEIGHTS BUT LITTLE EXPERIENCE ON THE BALL	5 LB/2 KG	7 LB/3 KG	10 LB/4 KG
EXPERIENCE WITH WEIGHTS AND BALL TRAINING	7 LB/3 KG	10 LB/4 KG	12-15 LB/5-6 KG

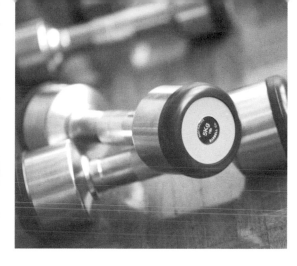

If you are used to strength training but not the exercise ball, do not be surprised if you need to go a little lighter when you first get on the ball. You will soon develop excellent core control and be able to build up the loads, and possibly even take it further.

If you find your muscles shaking or tensing, or you are holding your breath to complete reps, these are signs that you are compensating for the weakness of the muscle you are using. Change the load or adjust the degree of instability so that you feel you are moving with control.

Four ball workouts per week will help you reach your goals. Extra sessions are fine if you are sure to vary the programs and body areas worked. The training programs on page 181 are designed so that they can be done every day.

Take care
If an exercise causes you pain or feels uncomfortable, discontinue and seek advice from a health professional.

If you are unsure about your technique when exercising, a visit to a physical therapist or a respected personal trainer will be worthwhile.

GETTING STARTED

The magic of working out on a ball is its simplicity and ease of use.
This low cost, effective exercise option means you can train effectively anytime, anywhere.

All you need is:

> A good quality, correctly-sized exercise ball.
> A well-ventilated space that is free of sharp objects.
> A clear wall space.
> A non-slip surface or yoga mat.
> Hand weights; a few different levels of weights. See page 18.
> Two or three exercise bands of different strengths.
> Comfortable clothes.
> Non-slip exercise shoes.

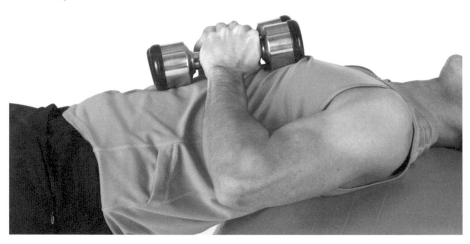

ALL ABOUT BALLS

Investing in a quality ball is important for its longevity and your comfort and safety. Choose a ball that has a non-slip surface and is burst-resistant, which means if punctured it will deflate slowly, not pop like a balloon.

The ideal ball, when properly inflated has you sitting with your hips level with or just slightly higher than your knees. Lower than this is more challenging to maintain good posture and any higher compromises your positioning in the prone position over the ball.

Inflate your ball to the point of firmness with a slight give. Use anything that will blow up an airbed or large inflatable toy; hand pumps, foot pumps and compressors all work well. Do not over-inflate your ball. If it is tight as a drum it may be uncomfortable and it will probably stretch. It is ideal to inflate a new ball to 75 percent capacity, leave it for a day or two to "relax," then fill it up to firm with a little give before you use it. Keep your ball away from extreme temperature changes and sharp objects.

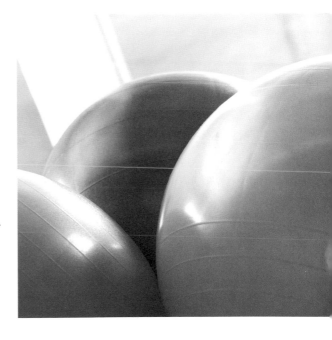

HAND WEIGHTS

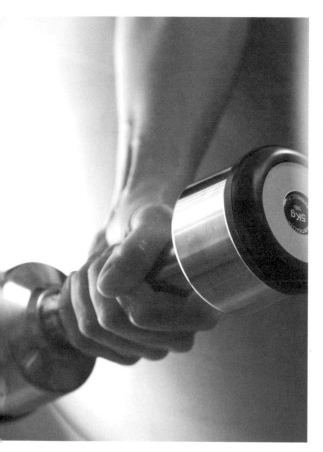

Hand weights are used in some exercises and can be used as alternatives to the band options. Hand weights ranging from 2 lbs to 10 lbs can be used on the ball depending on previous experience and strength. Use the table on page 18 as a guide. If you are used to weights, but not the ball, do not be surprised if you need to decrease the loads initially while you attain stability and balance on the ball.

RESISTANCE BANDS

Resistance bands provide an effective and convenient alternative to hand weights. They are inexpensive, light and easy to transport. Bands available in sporting and department stores range from a simple piece of elastic to a more sophisticated band with handle. They are color-coded indicating levels of load. The correct band will have you feeling like you're working but able to maintain technique up to the final repetition. If you are struggling, lengthen your band slightly, choose a lighter one or decrease the number of repetitions if you are struggling. Hand weights can be used as an alternative in all the band exercises described.

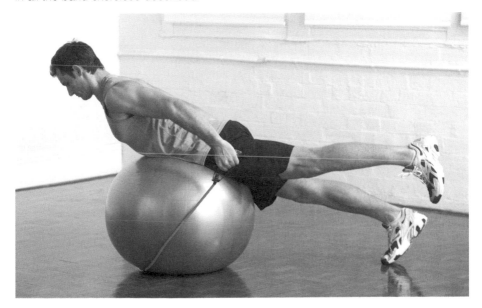

PERFECT POSTURE

Postural and movement awareness are the key elements in the ability to staying injury-free and being able to exercise and move with perfect form.

By becoming attuned to how you are moving and holding your body you can really optimize your training benefits.

Regularly run your mind through the following body set-up for perfect posture to finetune your form and move with finesse.

Head, neck and shoulders

Keep your neck long, light and in line with your spine.
Be sure that your chin is not poking forward or tilting towards your chest.
Avoid tensing and shrugging your neck and shoulders as this can lead to pain and possible injury. Monitor your neck and shoulders for ideal posture; shoulders rolled gently back and down, away from your ears, leaving your neck feeling long but relaxed.

Upper back

Hold your chest up and open as though showing off a priceless necklace.
Avoid the common temptation to drop your shoulders down and forward, which rounds your upper back. Elongate your spine and gently settle your shoulder blades down and inwards.

Natural lumbar curve

The spine is at its best when the natural curves are present. Aim to maintain the slight lumbar curve of your lower back by engaging your deep abdominals. Make sure that you have not exaggerated the curve or flattened or rounded out that area.

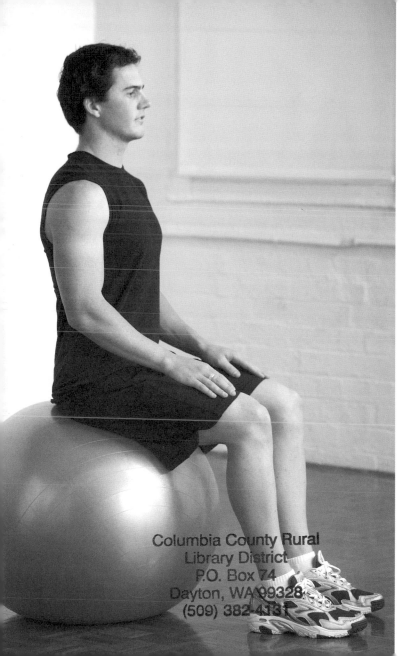

Columbia County Rural
Library District
P.O. Box 74
Dayton, WA 99328
(509) 382-4131

Seated body posture

Sit tall on the ball with your feet slightly forward so that the ball is not resting on your calves. You should be able to see your toes in front of your knees.

Sitting on your sit bones, elongate your spine to grow tall but without tension.

Make sure your natural lumbar curve is present and lightly draw in your lower abdomen to engage your deep abdominals. Settle your shoulders gently back and down.

ENGAGING
THE ABS AND CORE

The deep muscles around the shoulder girdle and lower back are important for control, injury prevention and fine form.

Core stability – what is it?

Core control is the ability of specific deep muscles to support the spine, shoulder girdle or pelvis. Healthy deep abdominal and back muscles contract to stabilize the lumbar vertebra and support virtually every movement you make. Without adequate stability from these muscles the risk of injury increases.

Your ticket to core stability

Sit tall and be aware of the natural curve in your lower back. Place one hand below your navel. Here, under your outer abs, lies your deepest abdominal group, the transversus abdominis or TA. This muscle works closely with other deep muscles such as multifidus, the diaphragm and pelvic floor to create a cylinder of stability around your lumbar spine.

Engaging the core

Gently draw your lower abdomen towards your lower back. The movement may feel very subtle or non-existent at first. Avoid sucking in your ribs or outer abdominals.

Relax your shoulders and continue to breathe normally. You may feel your pelvic floor lift as you engage your core abdominals as the muscles work together.

Persevere with this gentle drawing in of your lower abdomen. You will soon become more aware of the muscles working.

With practice, you should be able to engage your core before and during any activity.

Settle your shoulders

Shrugging or tensing your shoulders is a common compensation when people are stressed, overworked or struggling with an exercise. It is important to relax your neck and shoulders and learn to use the muscles that help settle the shoulders back and inwards into a healthy posture.

Sitting tall, gently glide your shoulder blades down and inward towards your tailbone. Keep your neck and shoulders relaxed as you set your shoulder blades into this "soft V" position.

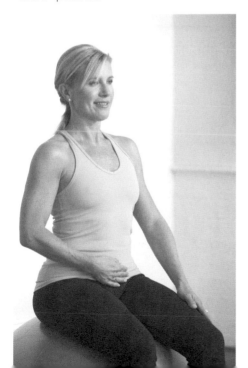
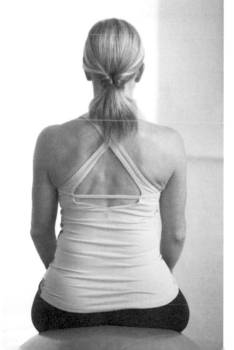

QUALITY
NOT QUANTITY

For injury-free, quality training and great results, there is nothing more important than good form.

Choosing an inappropriate exercise or progression, working out too heavily or too fast, or over-challenging your balance or stability will make an exercise ineffective or, worse still, unsafe.

Listen to your body and monitor your form

Pushing on regardless or "no pain no gain" only cheats your body. This approach devalues your training and reinforces bad movement patterns and habits.

You should expect to feel your muscles working (and be pleased when the last repetition is done) but be able to complete that last rep with the same control and quality as the first one.

Postural and movement awareness are a key focus of *Get on the Ball for Great Abs*. Always be conscious of your body alignment and suitable muscle use.

The signs of compensation for loss of control and form are:

> Activateing other muscles to get through the exercise. Bracing outer abdominals, squeezing thigh muscles, tensing neck and shoulders, tightening fists, curling toes and raising eyebrows are all signs.

> Shaking or movement where movement should not be occurring.

> Holding your breath.

> Loss of upright posture and natural spinal curves.

> The ball wobbling or moving unexpectedly.

Always work in harmony

Working strength, stability and balance together reaps the best results. Refer to the "Perfect Posture" on page 24 as often as you need to remind yourself of the all important position and technique hints for fabulous form and perfect posture.

It's not what you do, it's the way that you do it

BALL BASICS

Get on the Ball for Great Abs builds upon the following fundamental exercises which are described in full in *Get on the Ball*.

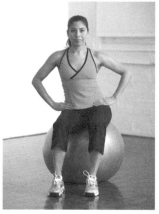

1. Seated mobility
Sitting tall on the ball, gently circling the hips or rounding and lengthening your back are simple warm-up moves.

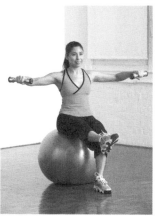

2. Seated stability and strength
Many upper body exercises, such as biceps curls, shoulder press, triceps press, can be performed sitting on the ball. Add a stabilizing challenge by raising one foot while maintaining good posture and control.

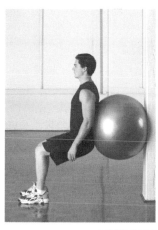

3. Wall squat

Squatting with the ball between your lower back and wall is a great thigh workout. Use your core to maintain a long, straight back as you roll the ball up and down the wall.

4. Ball as a bench/supine on the ball

Rolling down so that your head, neck and shoulders are on the ball and your feet are under your knees is an alternative to lying on a bench to perform chest press, flys or lateral pullovers. You will notice that your muscles work more on the ball, especially your gluteals and stabilizers.

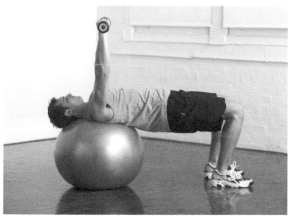

BALL BASICS

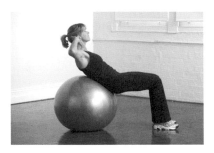

5. Abdominal curls

Lying with your lower back on the ball is a popular position for training abdominal muscles. If you're an ab curl pro you'll love the fresh challenge on the ball.

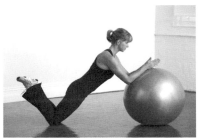

6. Roll away

The roll away works the inner and outer abdominals, laterals and more. Lean on the ball through your forearms, roll off your knees to your thighs to challenge inner and outer muscles simultaneously. Keep your shoulders back and down and engage your deep abdominals to prevent your back from swaying.

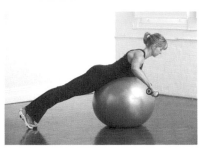

7. Prone on the ball

Lying on your back on the ball provides the ideal position for back and butt strengthening. A range of arm and leg options are selected to focus on upper or lower posterior strength.

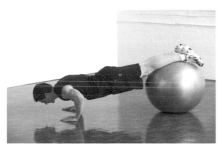

8. Push-ups

Perfomring push-ups on a ball requires extra stability and control. The further you walk out, the harder it will be. Make sure you keep your back straight and strong.

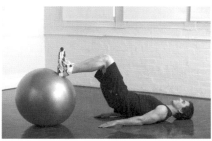

9. Hamstring roll

Lift your back off the floor and rolling the ball towards you, keeping just your heels on the ball, to challenge hamstring strength and spinal stability. It's even harder with your arms off the ground.

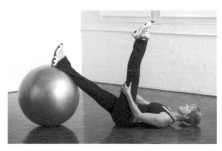

10. Flexibility

Stretches keep your muscles supple and your movement free and easy.

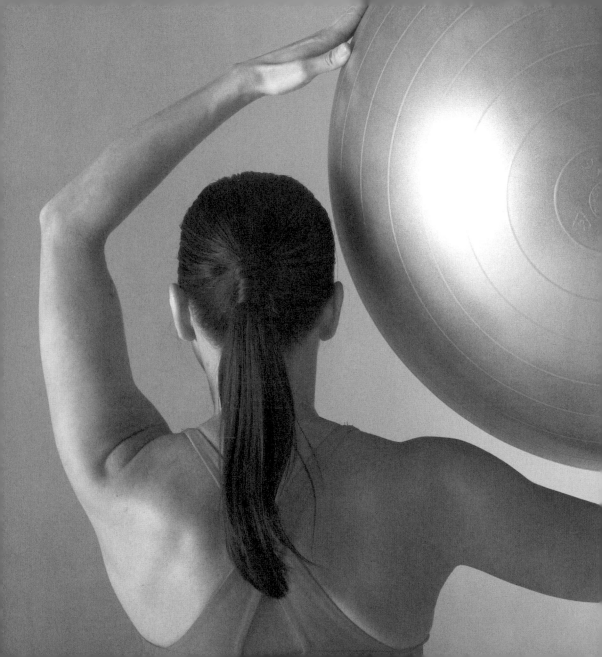

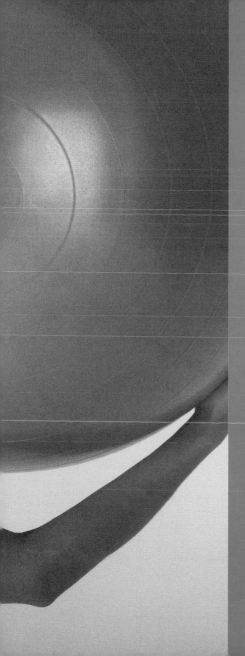

Warm-up, release tension and tightness

Gentle mobility moves prepare your body
for exercise, ease muscle tension, improve
postural awareness, assist joint mobility
and encourage graceful body movement,
not to mention relieving any discomfort
related to stiffness or tightness
in your body.

If you're new to ball fitness, or are getting
into shape after pregnancy these are
ideal exercises to help you become
familiar with the style of exercise and
find your comfort zone.

If you you have back issues these
options are just what your body needs.

The following exercises are also a fabulous
addition for those already working hard
on strength and stability.

EASE INTO ACTION

SEATED MOBILITY

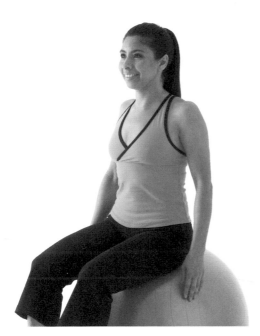

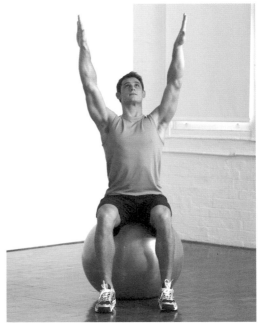

shoulder rolls

> Sit tall on the ball with your feet resting in front, hip-width apart.

> Elongate your spine.

> Breathe in as you roll your shoulders up, back and exhale as you settle them gently down and inwards.

> Repeat x 5

arm circles

> Breathe in as you reach your arms up, past the midline of your body.

> Exhale to arc them down, out and back to beside your hips.

> Repeat x 5

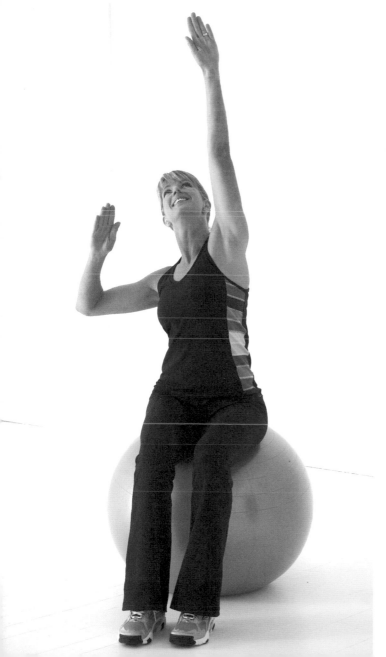

climb the ladder

> Sit tall on the ball and extend your arms upwards.
> Reach one arm, then the other, towards the sky, as though climbing a ladder.
> Allow the ball to roll slightly side to side.
> 10 reps each side.

SEATED
MOBILITY

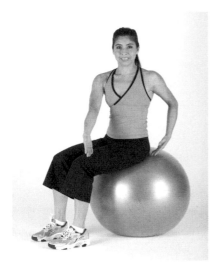

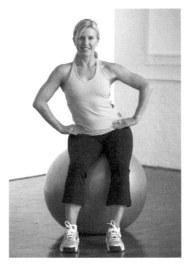

waist warm-up

> Sit with your feet hip width apart, elongate your
spine and relax your shoulders gently back and
down.

> Lightly draw in below the navel to engage your
core.

> Rotate your upper body side to side, reaching
alternate hands past the opposite knee. Keep
your legs and the ball still while you rotate above
the waist.

> Repeat x 5 each side, then sit tall and hold your
hand to the opposite knee for 5 breaths before
repeating the stretch to the other side.

pelvic clock

> Sit tall on the ball. Imagine your tailbone is the
center of a clock face.

> Gently roll the ball forward, rounding your lower
back, to 12 o'clock.

> Roll back, to slightly exaggerate the natural lumbar
curve, to 6 o'clock.

> Come back to the center then roll to each side
to 3 o'clock and 9 o'clock.

> Focus on lumbar mobility while you keep the
upper body and shoulders still and the movement
smooth.

> Repeat x 3 to 5.

> For variety roll your hips in a circle each
way or create a flowing figure 8.

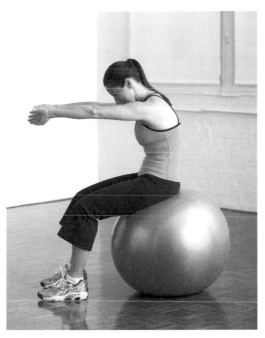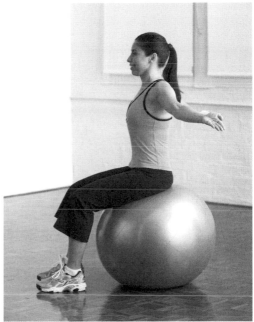

upper back warm-up

> Sit tall on the ball. Raise your arms sideways to shoulder height.

> Bring your hands forward, thumbs down, to meet in front of your chest.

> Feel your shoulder blades glide forward on your ribs as you round your upper back.

> Turn your palms upwards, sit tall and take your arms wide again.

> Repeat x 5

ROLLING
SIDE TO SIDE

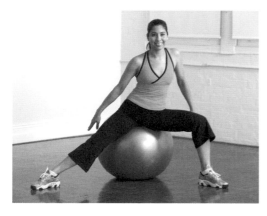

rolling side to side

> Sit upright and slightly forward on the ball, with your feet wide.

> Roll the ball from side to side, straightening and bending alternate knees.

> You can then add the following three arm actions:

shoulder roll

> Roll one shoulder up, back and down as you move to the side. Repeat on the other side.

> Rep x 5 each side

alternate arm circles

> Circle your arm forward, reaching up and arc it around and down in the direction you are rolling on the ball.

> Rep x 5 each side

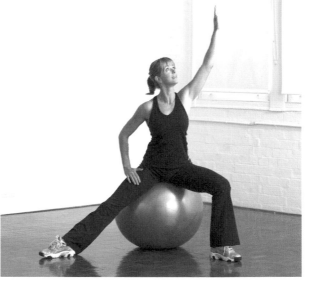

reach across

> Sweep your arm in a horizontal arc, out forward and across your body, towards the direction you are rolling the ball.
> You may want to rest your other hand on your bent knee for support.
> It is as though you are wiping a large table, really reaching out to the furthest side.
> Feel the rotation in your trunk and the stretch behind your shoulder blade.
> Rep x 5 each side

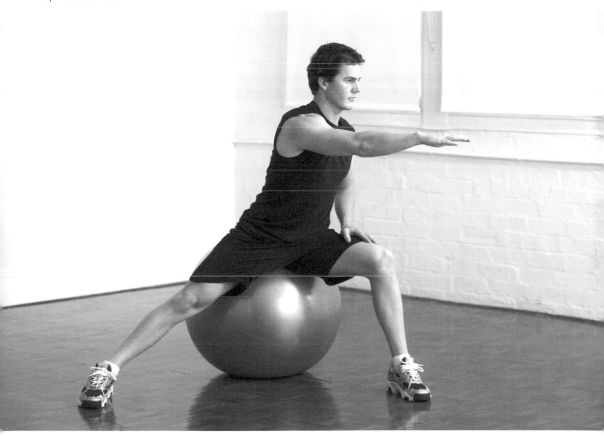

KNEELING MOBILITY

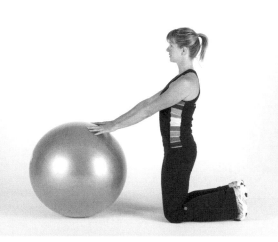

kneeling back and shoulder roll

Shoulder blade glide

> Kneel upright with the ball in front of you and reach your arms out to rest on the top of the ball.

> Roll the ball forward, tuck your chin in, and round your upper back gently.

> Roll back to upright kneeling, settling your shoulders back and down to finish.

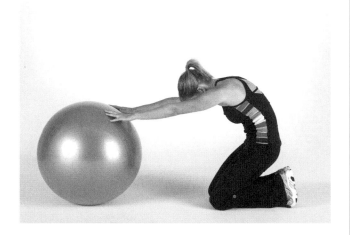

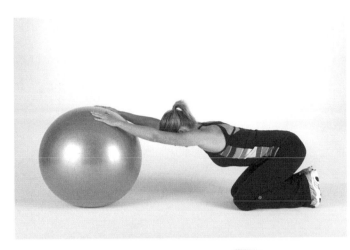

Spine roll

> Push the ball further forward this time as you sit back on your heels.

> Keep your spine straight as you stretch from your fingers to your hips.

> Roll slowly back up, one vertebra at a time.

> Starting by tucking your tailbone under, sequentially roll up, through your spine, finishing in an upright kneeling position, to once again settle your shoulders back and down.

> Sequence the shoulder blade glide and spine roll together.

> Rep x 5

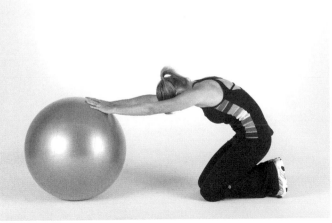

STANDING
MOBILITY

standing tall

> Stand with your feet hip-width apart, weight evenly spread through from heels to toes.

> Hold the ball in front, keep your arms relaxed.

> Soften your knees.

> Elongate your spine as though your are increasing the distance between each vertebra to grow taller.

> Settle your shoulders softly down and back, and gently lengthen your neck to hold your head high.

> Lightly draw in your abdomen, just below your navel to engage your core.

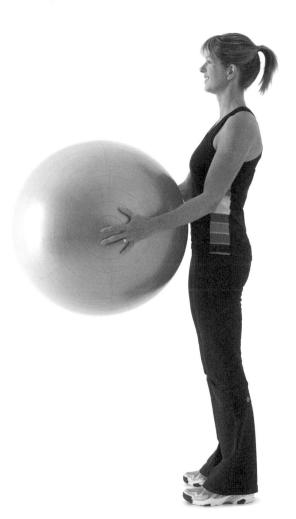

circle and reach

> Inhale as you circle the ball, forward and upward, towards the sky to stretch from head to toe.

> Exhale and lower the ball in front of your body to the resting position.

> Rep x 5

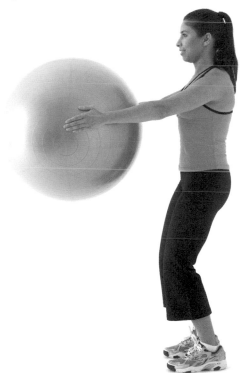

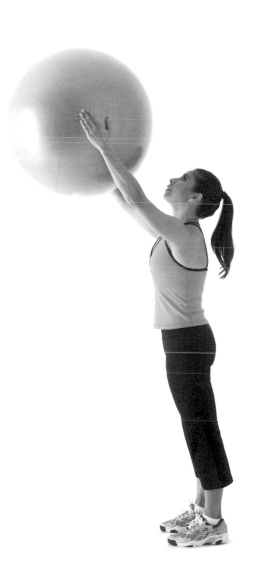

STANDING MOBILITY

reach and sit

> Stand tall, with your feet hip-width apart, and hold the ball in front of your body.

> Move the ball forward and reach as you sit down into a narrow squat position. Your spine leans forward, but remains long, strong and straight.

> Take your weight back into your heels, as you squat. This action will protect your knees.

> You should be able to wriggle your toes.

> As you stand up, reach the ball high.

> Rep x 10

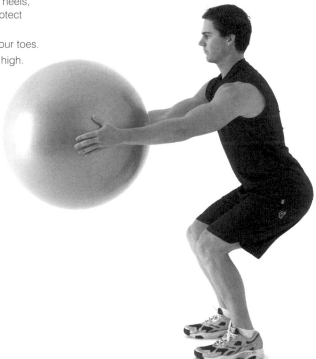

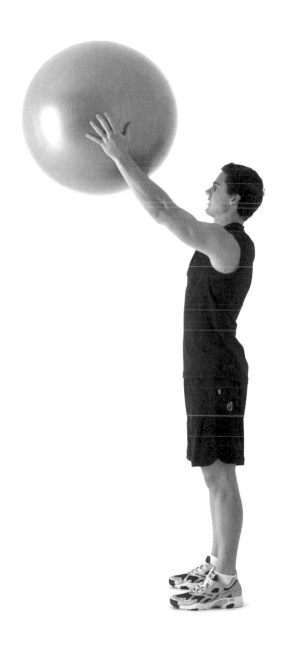

STANDING MOBILITY

standing back roll

> Stand with your feet wide and knees bent, with your fingers resting on the ball in front of you.

> Settle your shoulders and engage your deep abdominals by gently drawing in below the navel.

> Rolling the ball away, lean forward from the hips and direct your tailbone backwards, to stretch from your fingers to your hips.

> Increase the bend in your knees and keep your back straight as you reach forward.

> Curl to an upright stance, starting at your tailbone and rolling smoothly up, one vertebra at a time. Settle your shoulders back and down and stand tall to finish.

> Rep x 4

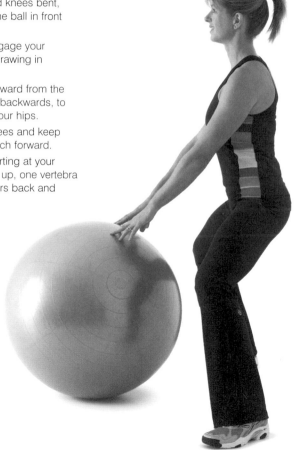

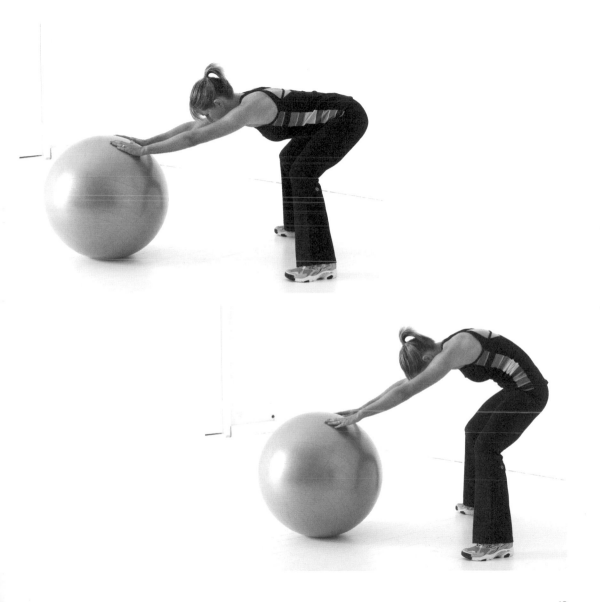

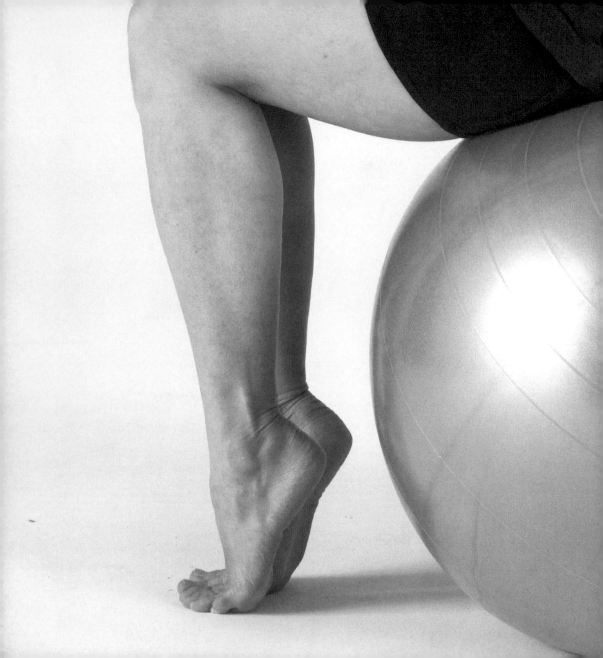

Balance and stability for a healthy back and fine form

Sitting on the ball is an excellent position to train for balance and core stability, as well as a proud posture and a healthy back.

Improved stabilization and balance will also enable you to take your athletic training, and performance to the next level.

Simple movements on the ball will challenge your ability to maintain the natural curvature of your spine, while keeping your body long and your shoulders relaxed.

In these exercises, you will learn to engage your deep abdominals to help keep your body and the ball stable as you challenge this control with various arm and leg movements.

As you improve, add asymmetrical movements and decrease your base of support to progress the challenge and further finetune your control. For example, bring your feet together, or lift one foot off the ground.

These low-impact stepping moves on the ball also serve as ideal exercise alternatives for post-pregnancy workouts or people looking for gentle exercise.

Regardless of your level of fitness, awareness and control of the deep abdominal stabilizing muscles are essential for a healthy back and body.

SEATED CORE CONTROL

SEATED CORE CONTROL

long, strong and stable

Starting position for all of the seated core exercises.

> Sit tall on the ball with your feet hip-width apart,
  heels directly under your knees.

> Be sure that your calves are not touching
  the ball.

> Arms should be relaxed and down by
  your sides.

> Lengthen your spine and relax your
  shoulders back and down.

> Draw in the muscles below your navel
  to engage your deep abdominals.

seated walk

Action

Step forward and back

> Slowly walk one step forward and back.

> Keep your body upright and maintain a neutral
  lumbar curve as the ball rolls.

> Avoid rocking your pelvis from side to side.

> Rep x 10

Decrease the challenge

> Lift your heel or foot alternately without
  stepping forward.

Increase the challenge

> Walk two steps forward

> As you walk forward and back, add arm circles
  that move up and out, as though you are
  swimming to the surface.

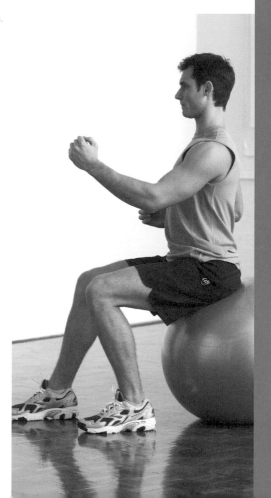

SIDE STEP

sideways stability

Action

Step up and over

> Lift your right foot out to the side, then step your left foot across, bringing your feet together.

> From this position, repeat the step to the left.

> Continue stepping from side to side, keeping your shoulders relaxed and your back straight and strong.

> Keep your torso upright as the ball and your body travel side to side; don't lean.

> Reps x 10 in each direction

Decrease the challenge

> Side tap only (page 54) without the step across.

> Take a smaller step across.

> Keep your hands resting on the ball.

Increase the challenge

> Step across and lift the second foot without placing it on the ground.

> Add single arm lateral raise on the side you are stepping towards.

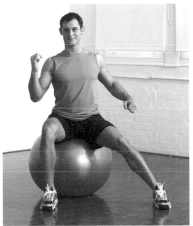

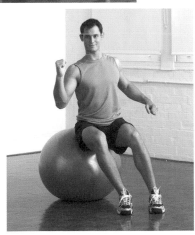

SIDE TAP

lateral control

Action
Tap your foot to the side

> Keeping your knee bent, tap one foot lightly out to the side.
> Raise both your arms sideways as you tap each leg.
> Return to the center.
> Keep your waist long, your body upright and the ball still.
> Reps x 10 on one side then the other or alternate from side to side.

Decrease the challenge
> Lift your foot just off the floor.
> Or tap just a little out from the starting point.
> Keep your hands resting lightly on the ball.

Increase the challenge
> Adding arm action on the same side further challenges control.
> Raise your arm sideways to shoulder height.
> This is harder still by holding a light weight in your hand.

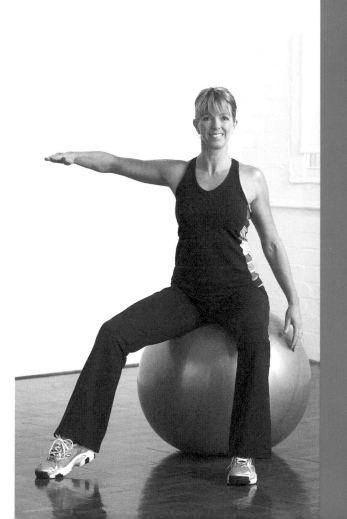

ROTATE AND CONTROL

feel your waist working as you challenge your stability

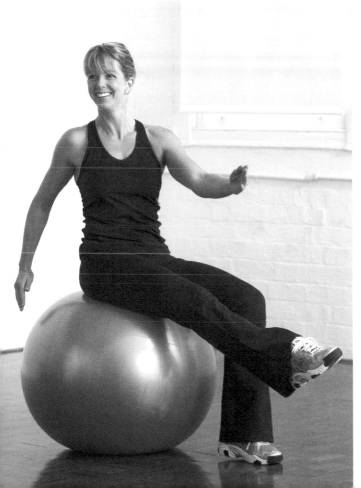

Action

Rotate and lift

> Sit tall, lengthen your waist and draw inwards below your navel.

> Rotate your upper body to the right reaching across with your left arm.

> Simultaneously lift your right foot just off the floor.

> Rotate from side to side, lifting the leg on the side to which you are turning.

> Use your core to keep your pelvis, legs and the ball still.

Decrease the challenge

> Perform the rotation without the leg lift.

> Lift your heel, leaving your toe on the floor.

> Perform the leg lift without the rotation.

Increase the challenge

> Extend your knee so your raised leg is straight.

> Close your eyes.

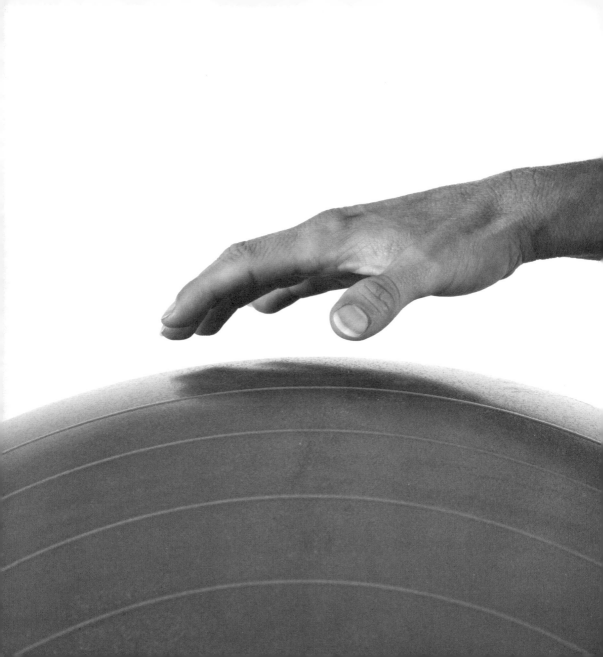

An upbeat warm-up to really get you moving

These exercises are not only fun, you'll also be surprised by the energetic workout

Combining low-impact moves while bouncing the ball warms up your upper and lower body. Ball bouncing is fun, but don't be misled, the benefits of these warm-ups and the cardiovascular options are invaluable.

When standing and bouncing the ball, maintain a connection with your core muscles and monitor your posture regularly.

Keep your upper body straight and strong. Bend your knees not your back.

Avoid shrugging your shoulders by focusing on keeping your shoulder blades set.

Your wrists must stay strong. Bounce the ball with your fingertips rather than smacking it with your your palms.

Really put some energy into the bounce. You'll get a great warm-up that will make you feel fantastic.

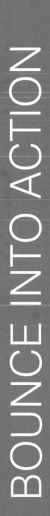

BOUNCE INTO ACTION

STEP AND BOUNCE

put a spring in your step

Starting position
> Stand with your feet together, holding the ball in front of your body.
> Engage your deep abdominals. Make sure your spine is long and shoulders are relaxed.

Action
Step from side to side and bounce the ball
> Bend your knees as you step from side to side.
> Bounce and catch the ball as you step.

Decrease the challenge
> Step from side to side without the ball or stand still in a wide squat and bounce the ball.

Increase the challenge
> Increase the speed.
> Try stronger bouncing of the ball.

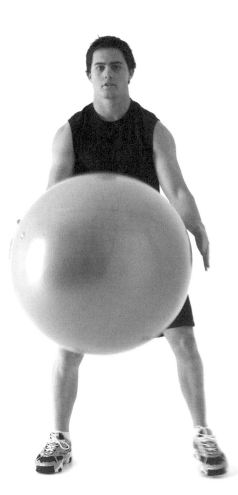

TRAINER TIPS

BEND YOUR KNEES, NOT YOUR BACK.

KEEP YOUR UPPER BODY TALL.

TO REALLY WARM-UP YOUR ARMS, BOUNCE THE BALL HIGH.

CONTROL THE KNEE YOU STAND ON AND MAKE SURE YOU ARE NOT LOCKING IT STRAIGHT.

AVOID SLOUCHING FORWARD.

KEEP YOUR CHEST UP AND YOUR DEEP ABDOMINALS ENGAGED.

CURL
SWING

warm up your shoulders and thighs

Starting position
> Stand with your feet wide, holding the ball in front of your body.

Action

Curl and swing

> Bend your knees, swing the ball to one side, as you step onto your right foot, swinging the ball to the same side.

> Lift the left leg and curl it behind you.

> Repeat to the other side.

Decrease the challenge
> Perform the move without the ball.

Increase the challenge
> Make the moves more energetic and perform a deeper squat as you swing through.

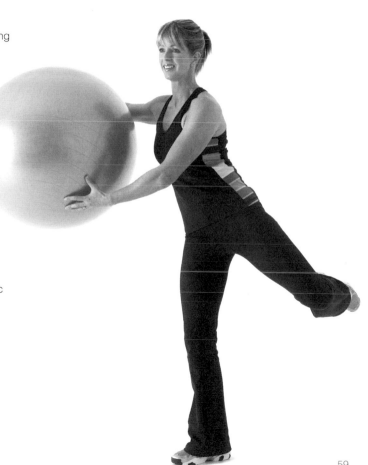

DOUBLE STEP
AND BOUNCE

follow the bouncing ball

Starting position
> Stand tall, with your feet together, holding the ball in front.
> Settle your shoulders down and activate your deep abdominals.

Action
Two steps sideways with a double bounce
> Take two steps sideways.
> Bounce the ball twice, keeping in sync with your stepping action.

Decrease the challenge
> Double step without the ball or stick with Step and Bounce on page 58

Increase the challenge
> Wider, deeper side steps.
> Stronger bounce.
> Increase the speed a little.

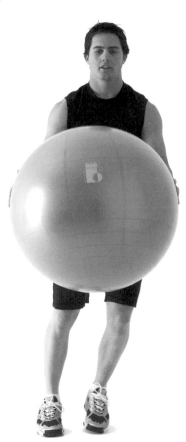

TRAINER TIPS

BOUNCE THE BALL SO YOU HAVE TO REACH UP TO CATCH IT.

BEND YOUR KNEES AS YOU STEP

KEEP THE CHEST UP AND AVOID LEANING FORWARD THE BALL.

KEEP YOUR BACK STRAIGHT.

BEND KNEES AT EACH END.

RAINBOW

reach for the sky

Starting position
> Standing tall, holding the ball.
> Abdominals set and shoulders relaxed.

Action
Two steps sideways, reaching the ball up and over
> Take two steps sideways.
> Arc the ball up and over your head and finish
  with the ball beside your hip. This is the
  end of the "rainbow."
> Reach tall through the middle of the move
  but bend your knees as you finish.

Decrease the challenge
> Perform the move without the ball.

Increase the challenge
> Add a small leap as you
  step through the middle
  of the sequence.
> Reach higher in the
  middle and bend your
  knees deeper at each
  end, taking your ball
  closer to the floor.

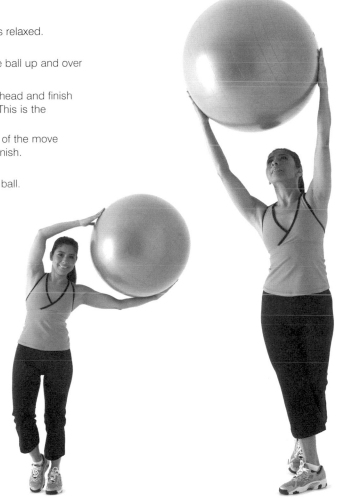

BOXER
BOUNCE

warm up your arms and work your waist

Starting position

> Stand in a wide-based squat, knees bent.

> Hold the ball in front of your abdomen.

> Lengthen your spine and engage your deep abdominals.

Action
Bounce and rotate

> Bounce the ball using both hands. Keep your wrists strong and bounce with your fingers, not your palms.

> Keeping the rhythm, change to bouncing the ball with one hand, then the other.

> Rotate through your waist as you bounce, reaching one arm forward and bending the other elbow back behind you.

> Keep your legs bent and still to make sure that your upper body rotates on a stable base.

Decrease the challenge

> Less rotation

> Waist warm-up on page 38.

Increase the challenge

> Increase the speed and rotation.

> Change to two bounces with each hand.

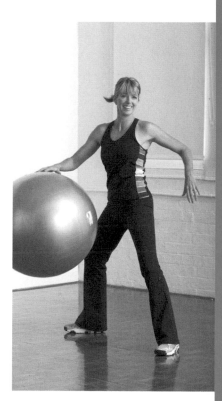

TRAINER TIPS

KEEP YOUR ELBOWS TUCKED IN CLOSE TO YOUR RIBS.

BE SURE THAT YOUR KNEES STAY BENT AND STILL.

THE ARM ACTION IS SIMILAR TO THAT USED WHEN RUNNING.

HOLD YOUR CHEST UP HIGH.

KEEP YOUR BODY UPRIGHT.

THIS MOVE IS A LITTLE LIKE DRIBBLING A BASKETBALL.

SKIP AND
BOUNCE

get those feet moving

Starting position
> Stand with you feet hip-width apart,
  holding the ball in front of your hips.
> Deep abdominals are engaged and
  shoulders relaxed.

Action
Jog from foot to foot as you bounce.

> Staying on the spot, skip from
  foot to foot.
> Bounce the ball with alternate hands.

Decrease the challenge
> Walk on the spot and bounce from
  hand to hand.

Increase the challenge
> Increase the energy and speed of
  the movement.
> Change from single to double
  as you skip and bounce on each side.
> Perform jumping jacks while bouncing
  the ball.

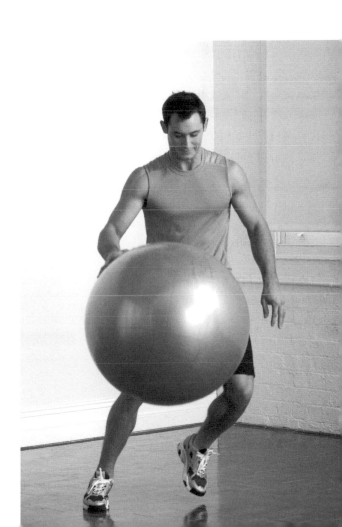

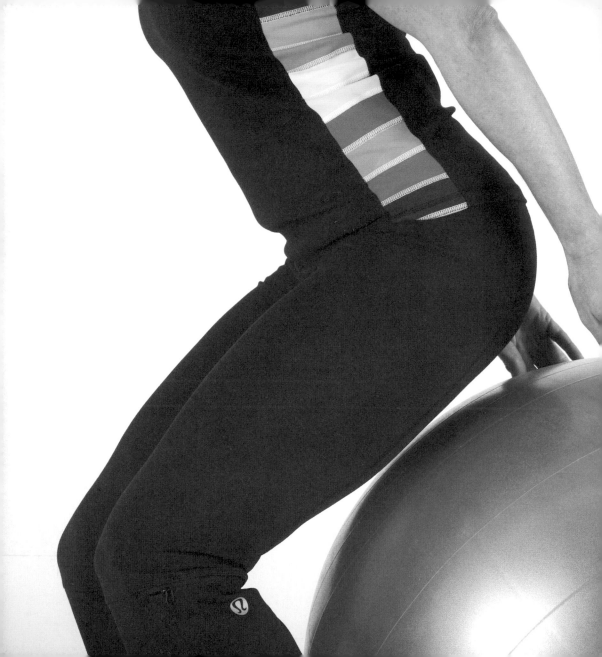

Bounce your way to
fitness and a fabulous core

The seated bounce is a fun, effective way to simultaneously improve your general fitness and core stability. Bouncing on the ball is a great alternative to other warm-ups and low- impact cardiovascular training. You'll feel your legs working and your heart pumping. It's enjoyable but it's harder than it looks.

Technique is important. Make sure you sit tall, keep your feet forward so your calves do not touch the ball, and your bottom stays in contact as you bounce.

Focus on perfect posture, keeping your spine long, neck and shoulders relaxed and deep abdominals switched on.

Perform each move for a minute or more and combine them for an effective 10-minute workout.

Note: If you have knee, neck, or back pain, seated bouncing is not for you. If this is the case, you can perform all the moves without the bounce. Decreased stress and increased focus on stability is exactly what you need.

SEATED BOUNCE

BASIC BOUNCE

fitness becomes child's play

Starting position for all
seated bounce exercises

> Sit tall on the ball, with your arms
  by your sides and your feet hip-
  width apart.

> Be sure your calves are not
  touching the ball and you can see
  your toes beyond your knees.

> Draw in the muscles below
  your navel to switch on your
  core abdominals.

> Relax your shoulders back
  and down.

Action
Bounce and reach

> Bounce up and down on the ball.

> Reach forward and backwards as
  you bounce, bending your elbows
  on the way back.

Decrease the challenge

> Keep your hands resting on
  the ball.

> Decrease the bounce intensity.

> March in place without bouncing.

Increase the challenge

> Increase the bounce intensity.

> Try alternating running arms.

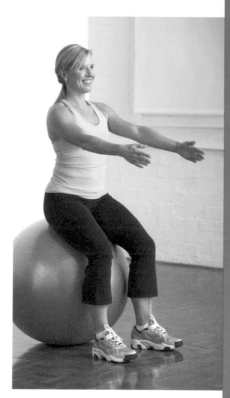

TRAINER TIPS

KEEP THE WEIGHT
IN YOUR HEELS TO
PROTECT YOUR KNEES.

BE SURE YOUR BACK
STAYS LONG
AND STRONG.

KEEP CONTACT
BETWEEN YOUR
BOTTOM AND THE BALL.

IF YOU FEEL
DISCOMFORT PERFORM
THE MOVE WITHOUT
THE BOUNCE.

HEELS
FORWARD

control your body while you bounce

Starting position
> As for Basic Bounce.

Action
Alternate heel tap forward as you bounce.

> Begin with a comfortable bounce rhythm, keeping both feet on the floor.
> Add an alternating heel tap on the floor. Take one heel forward and back, then the other.
> Reach your arms forward and back, bending your elbows on the way back.

Decrease the challenge
> Heel tap forward without the bounce to focus on stability and balance.
> Leave your hands resting on the ball beside you.

Increase the challenge
> Alternate your arm action so you reach forward with the same arm as the moving heel.
> Reach both or alternate your arms towards the ceiling.

Go harder
> Double-time heels. A faster alternating heel tap where one heel is moving forward as the other moves back. Opposite arm reach works well here.
> To really challenge balance and stability, take your foot forward but do not touch it to the floor in either the regular heel pattern or double-time version.

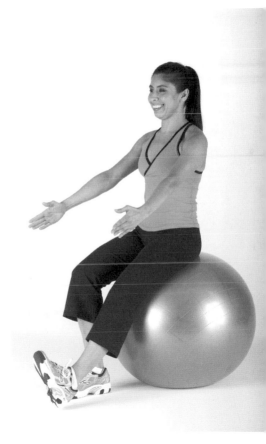

STAR
JUMPS

jumping jacks never felt so good

Starting position
> Sit tall on the ball, feet and knees together.
> Set your deep abdominals and draw your shoulders back and down.

Action

Jump out and in
> Jump your feet wide and back together.
> Raise your arms sideways as your feet jump out.

Decrease the challenge
> Without bouncing tap one foot and then the other to the side.
> Leave your hands resting on the ball beside your hips.

Increase the challenge
> Lift your knees higher as you jump out and in.
> Take your arms out sideways and up above your head.

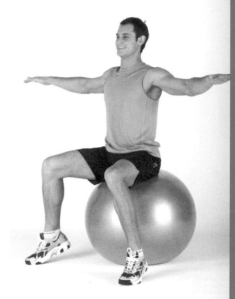

TRAINER TIPS

BE SURE YOU DO NOT LET YOUR LOWER BACK ROUND OR THE BALL ROLL FORWARD.

FOCUS ON KEEPING YOUR WAIST LONG AND YOUR UPPER BODY STRONG AND STABLE.

THE MOVEMENT HAPPENS FROM THE WAIST DOWN.

SKI JUMPS

stability, fitness and get fit to ski

Starting position
> Seated tall on the ball, feet together.
> Arms relaxed by your sides.
> Engage your core.

Action
Start with a basic bounce.
Jumping side to side.

> With your knees and feet together jump both feet to one side then the other.
> Do a double bounce on each side.
> As you jump to the right reach your left arm forward and draw your right elbow back by your side, then reverse the movement.

Decrease the challenge
> Keep your arms by your side.
> Step side to side without the bounce.

Increase the challenge
> Jump faster from side to side with a single bounce.
> For truly challenging core control hold your arms above your head.

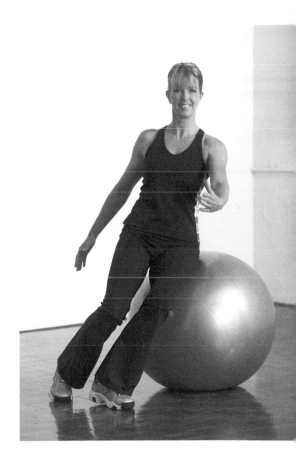

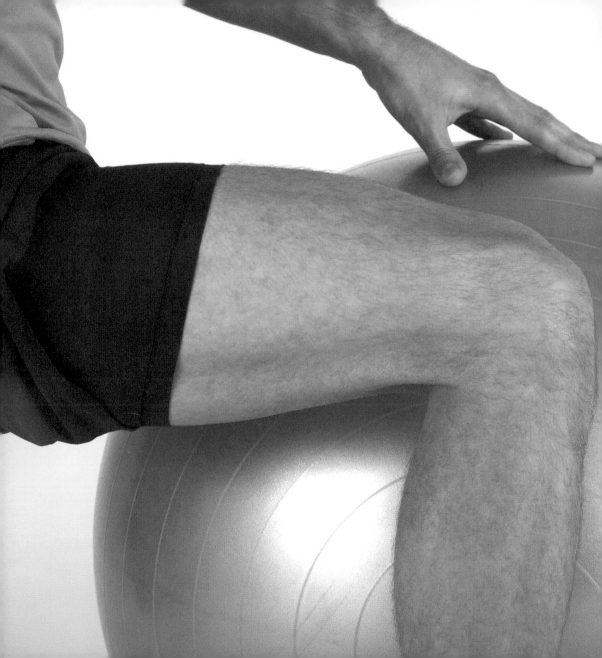

Stand tall for great abs, butt, and thighs

In additon to engaging the core, the following exercises hone in on strengthening quadriceps and gluteals with varying levels of balance and stability.

The single leg series provides some of the most challenging balance exercises in this book, whereas the ball-assisted lunge is easier than the regular non-ball version.

Whichever exercise you choose, you can expect to feel your legs working. Putting these exercises into your program means that toned thighs and a strong, taut derriere will soon be yours.

If your weak point is your knees concentrate on keeping the weight back in your heels and don't bend too deep. If you experience any knee pain, try the basic wall squat as described in ball basics on page 31.

To train your quads without any load through the knee, perform the seated leg raise from page 30.

STANDING STRENGTH

BALL-ASSISTED LUNGE

long lean legs, and a beautiful butt

Starting position
> Stand beside the ball with your feet together and your hand resting on the ball.
> Take a big step backwards with the leg that is closest to the ball.
> With both feet facing to the front, bend both your knees and lift your back heel off the floor.
> You should balance your weight through the heel of the front foot and the ball of the back foot.
> Incline your upper body slightly forward but keep your back straight, chest up and shoulders back.

Action
Lunge and lift
> Bend both knees further to lower your back knee towards the floor.
> Keep the ball by your hip. Try to avoid leaning into it for stability.
> 15 reps on each leg.

Decrease the challenge
> Perform only a shallow lunge or replace with seated leg raise, see page 30.
> 10 reps each side.

Increase the challenge
> Lunge deeper or increase the reps.

TRAINER TIPS

MAINTAIN AN EQUAL BALANCE OF WEIGHT IN BOTH FEET.

AVOID LEANING INTO THE BALL.

STRETCH

QUADS STRETCH (SEE PAGE 169)

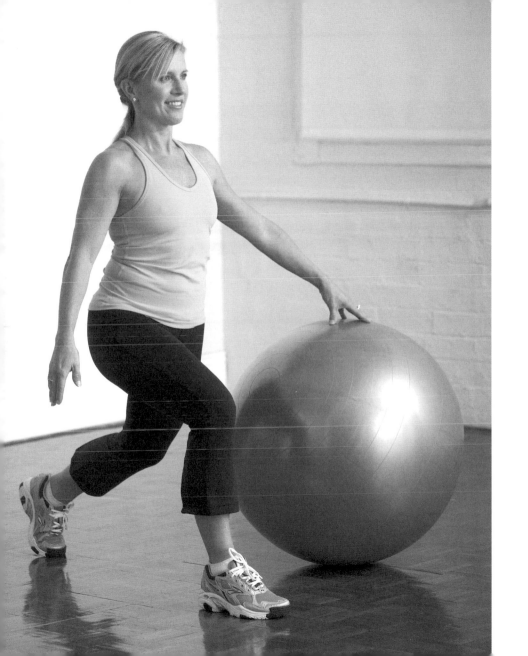

SINGLE
LEG LUNGE

strength, stretch and stability

An advanced strength and stability option that requires good balance and stability, quad strength and healthy knees.

Starting position

> Standing with the ball beside you, roll the ball back and "catch it" with the top of your foot.
> The ball should be under your shoelaces. It should be far enough back that your raised knee is behind you and the front of your hip is on slight stretch.
> Keep your body upright.
> The supporting leg must have a bent knee and the weight should be taken through your heel not your toes.
> Be sure your hips are level, and your pelvis and chest are facing forward. Do not let your body rotate to one side.

Action

Bend and stand

> Bend your front knee into a slight squat, keeping the weight in that heel.
> Lean your raised foot slightly into the ball as it rolls back.
> Push through your heel to stand back up but avoid locking the knee.
> 15 reps on each leg.

Decrease the challenge

> Use the wall or a chair to assist your balance.
> Do the ball-assisted lunge on page 72.
> 5 to 10 reps on each leg.

Increase the challenge

> Add upright row: Using level 2 or 3 hand weights, start with them on either side of your front knee. Raise the weights to chest height as you stand and lower the weights as you lunge.

TRAINER TIPS

KEEP THE WEIGHT
IN HEEL OF THE FOOT
ON THE FLOOR.

KEEP YOUR PELVIS
SQUARE TO THE FRONT.

FOCUS ON FORM AND
CORE CONTROL.

STRETCH

QUADS STRETCH
(SEE PAGE 169)

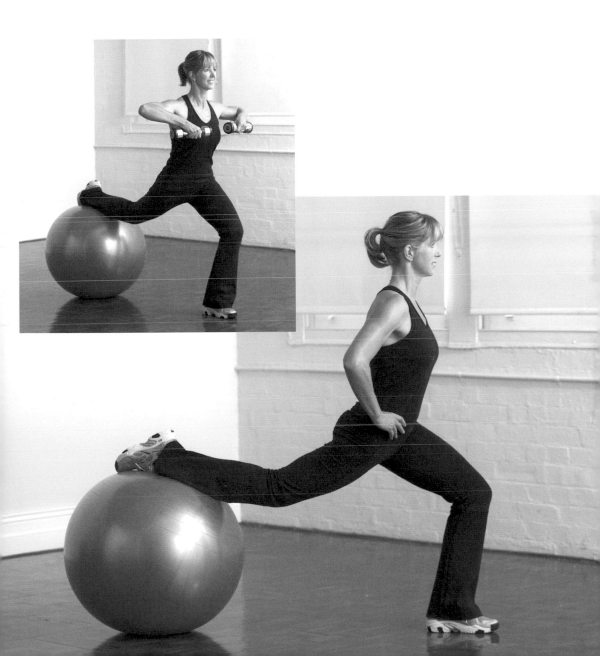

LEAN
AND LIFT

thighs to die for

This is an advanced exercise for strength and control and is not for the faint-hearted.

Starting position

> With the ball placed in front of you. Stand with your feet hip width apart and knees bent.

> Lean forward from your hips to rest your hands lightly on the ball.

> Roll your shoulders back and down. Engage your deep abdominals and be sure that your spine is straight.

> Extend one leg behind you, resting your foot on the floor.

> Shift your weight back into the heel of your front foot. This will protect your knee.

Action

Raise and lower

> Be sure your front knee is bent and the weight is in your heel.

> Slowly raise and lower your back leg, keeping it straight and strong.

> Make sure your core is engaged and you breathenormally.

> In this long, strong position, rest your hands lightly on the ball. The less you lean, the more you will strengthen. As you raise your leg, reach your opposite arm up and forward. Aim to lengthen from your fingers to your toes.

> 15 reps on each side.

Decrease the challenge

> Do the ball-assisted lunge on page 72.

> Keep both hands on the ball.

> Raise your foot off the floor just a little.

> Decrease the reps.

Increase the challenge

> Hold the long, strong position for 3 breaths each time you raise your arm and leg.

> Hold your leg up straight and draw 5 small leg circles with your foot, moving in first a clockwise direction, followed by an anti-clockwise direction.

> Bend your supporting leg even further.

TRAINER TIPS

IT IS ESSENTIAL TO KEEP YOUR SUPPORTING KNEE BENT.

KEEP THE RAISED LEG LONG AND STRONG.

FOR A GREAT BUTT WORKOUT SQUEEZE YOUR BACK LEG STRAIGHT.

MAKE SURE YOUR BODY AND PELVIS ARE SQUARE TO THE FLOOR.

STRETCH

QUADS STRETCH (SEE PAGE 169)

POSTERIOR HIP STRETCH (SEE PAGE 173)

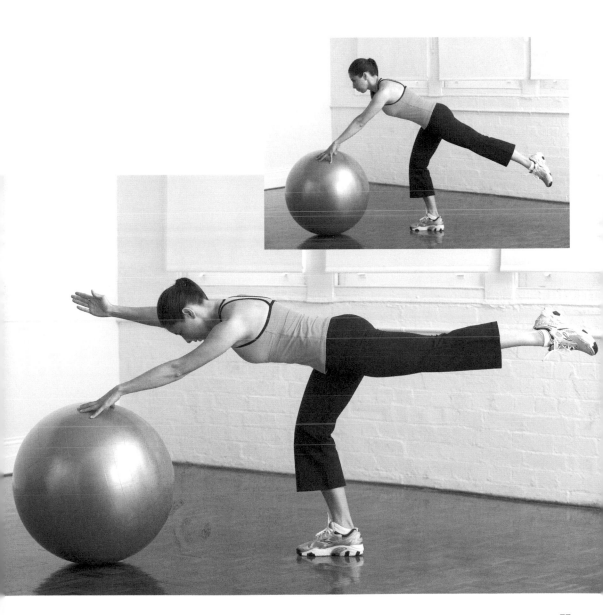

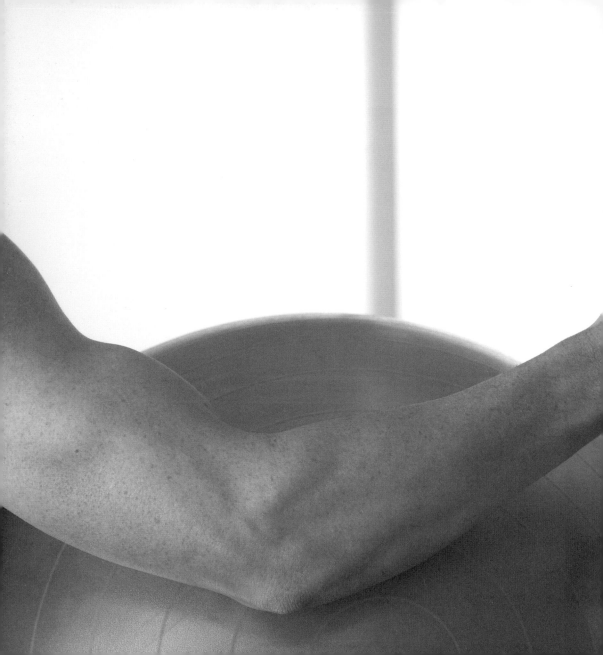

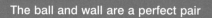

The ball and wall are a perfect pair

Ball and wall combinations provide effective training options for everyone. The following exercises range from gentle shoulder stabilization to new variations on an old favorite, the wall squat.

The wall provides gentle alternatives for moves that are normally performed on the ground such as the ball hover and push-up. Working at the wall is less intense than working on the floor against gravity, providing the ideal solution for people who need to take it easy.

These exercises are a great way to train for stability and strength.

AT THE WALL

WALL
WALK

roll and control

Starting position

> Stand with the ball between your lower back and the wall.

> Roll down to the "seated" position.

> Your back should be straight and parallel to the wall and your tailbone in contact with the ball.

> Drawing your lower abdomen towards the wall.

> You should be able to see your toes beyond your knees.

> Hold level 3 hand weights by your sides.

Action

Walk up the wall

> 'Walk up the wall' four steps and 'down the wall' four steps. Avoid leaning from side to side.

> Add alternating single arm bicep curls.

> 20 reps x 2 sets

Decrease the challenge

> Perform this exercise without weights.

> Wall squat. See page 31.

Increase the challenge

> Single leg wall squat: Place all your weight on one foot with the other foot resting lightly on the floor. Add a single arm bicep curl on the same side.

TRAINER TIPS

ROLL UP AND DOWN, BUT NOT SIDE TO SIDE.

KEEP YOUR WEIGHT IN YOUR HEELS TO PROTECT YOUR KNEES.

BE SURE YOU ARE NOT LEANING FORWARD OR BACK.

STRETCH TIP

QUADS STRETCH (SEE PAGE 169)

DO NOT LEAN INTO THE BALL.

THE BALL SHOULD ROLL UP AND DOWN THE WALL A LITTLE.

STRETCH

QUADS STRETCH (SEE PAGE 169)

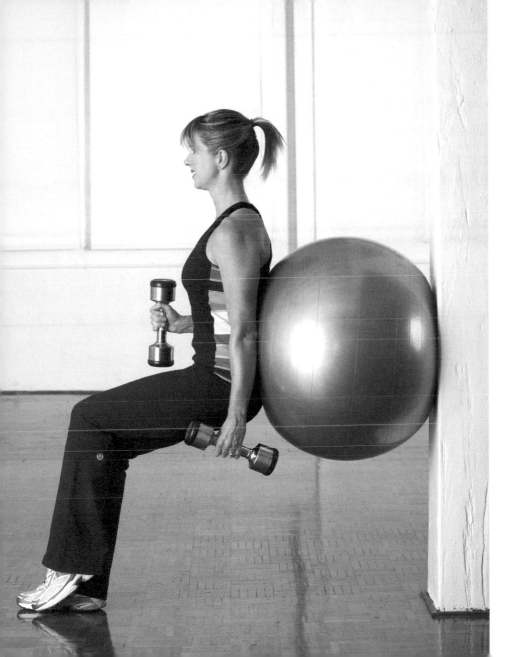

WALL HOVER

stability and control, less stress on your spine

A perfect alternative to the ball hover on the floor, this exercise improves strength and stability, without putting a load on the spine.

Starting position

> Stand at the wall with your forearms on the ball at chest height (you should be able to see over the top of the ball).

> Set your shoulder blades gently downward, and engage your deep abdominals. Lightly turn on your gluteals to stop your hips from bending.

> Take a step back with each foot.

Action

Lean and hold

> Leaning into your forearms, maintain straight, strong alignment from head to toe.

> Breathe as you make sure your shoulders are down, your back is straight and your hips are not bent. Hold for 5 slow breaths then step forward to relax.

> Repeat x 3

Decrease the challenge

Stand a little closer to the wall.

Increase the challenge

> Walk your feet further from the wall.

> Add a single leg raise. Raise one leg behind you and hold it straight and just off the floor. Keep your pelvis square to the wall.

> For more upper body control, hold your alignment as you roll the ball slightly from side to side.

TRAINER TIPS

MAINTAIN POSTURAL ALIGNMENT. AVOID ROUNDING YOUR UPPER BACK, ARCHING YOUR LOWER BACK AND BENDING AT THE HIPS.

STRETCH

WALL STRETCH
(SEE PAGE 178)

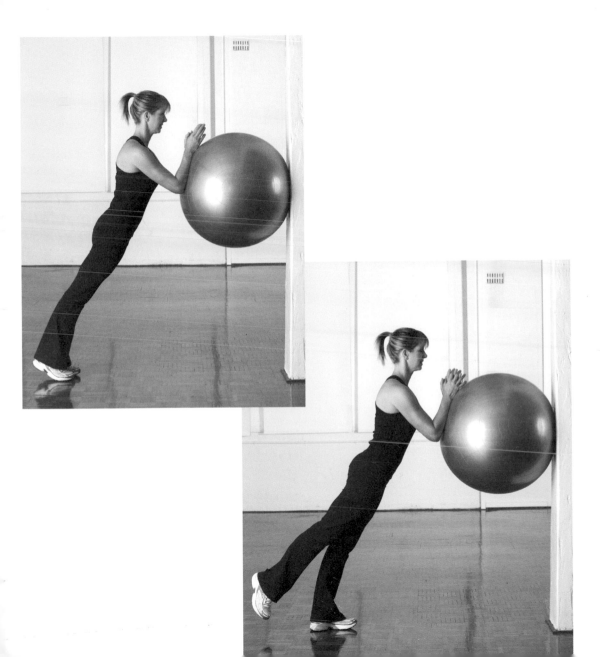

WALL
TRICEPS

stabilize your shoulders while you strengthen your arms

Starting position

> Stand upright with your arms outstretched, holding the ball against the wall, slightly below chest height.

> Arms shoulder width apart and elbows tucked in.

> Set your shoulders and core abdominals and step back from the wall.

Action

Bend your elbows and roll the ball

> Bend your elbows, lean inward and roll the ball slightly down the wall.

> Your arms glide close to your ribs as you lean in.

> Roll the ball up as you push back to straighten your arms.

> 15 x 2 sets

Decrease the challenge

> Stand closer to the wall.

Increase the challenge

> Start with the ball a little lower and walk feet further from the wall.

> Stand on one leg, holding the other leg just off the floor behind. Keep your pelvis square to the wall and avoid the temptation to rotate it to the raised leg side.

TRAINER TIPS

OBSERVE AND CORRECT FOR LOSS OF CONTROL SUCH AS SHOULDER SHRUG, ROUNDING UPPER BACK, SWAY IN LOWER BACK, OR BENDING AT THE HIPS.

STRETCH

WALL STRETCH (SEE PAGE 178)

SIDE STRETCH AND TRICEPS (SEE PAGE 174)

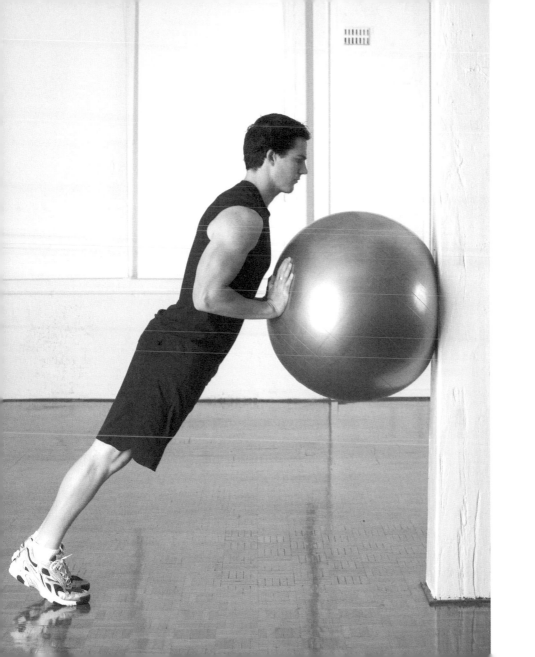

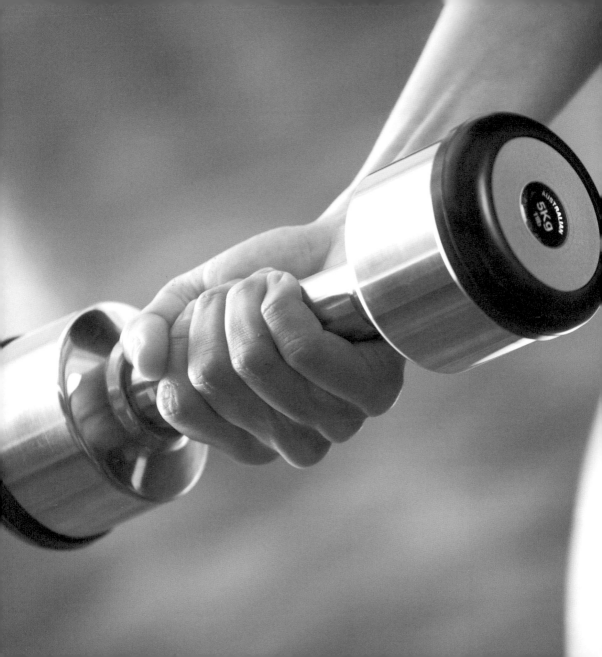

Strength and stability unite

Performing traditional strength moves while sitting on an unstable base has many benefits — fresh challenge, balance, stability and improved form.

Hand weights are an effective way of adding load to boost upper body strength and can be used in each of the following exercises, but for variety and convenience resistance bands are introduced in this section. Band and ball combinations provide equally effective training and are a practical alternative to hand weights for travellers and fitness fanatics on the move.

This section starts off with a surprising quads and butt workout that will have your thighs telling you they exist, followed by some fresh, effective upper body strength and stability exercises.

SEATED STRENGTH

SEATED
SEMI-SQUAT

a small move, a big workout

Starting position

> Sit slightly forward on the ball with your fingers resting by your hips.

> Feet out in front of the ball, hip-width apart.

> Heels on the floor, toes up.

> Elongate your spine, engage your abdominals and settle your shoulders downwards.

Action

Start to stand then change your mind

> Lean slightly forward to take the weight into your heels.

> Raise your bottom just a little off the ball.

> Keep both hands in contact with the ball, standing only as high as your arm length allows.

> Keep your chest up. Your head should be travelling up and down, not forward and back.

> 20 x 2 sets

Decrease the challenge

> Raise your bottom slightly, keeping in contact with the ball.

Increase the challenge

> To engage your inner thigh muscles by bringing your feet close and squeeze your knees together.

> Lower very slowly and just touch the ball lightly rather than sitting down each time. You'll feel it!

> Single leg load: Rest one foot lightly on the floor, using it for balance only while you stand and sit. Watch you don't lean sideways. 15 reps on each leg.

TRAINER TIPS

AVOID THE TEMPTATION TO TAKE A HAND OFF THE BALL AND LEAN TO ONE SIDE.

KEEP THE WEIGHT BACK IN YOUR HEELS.

THE SLOWER AND MORE GENTLY YOU SIT DOWN, THE TOUGHER THE WORKOUT.

STRETCH

HIP AND CHEST STRETCH (SEE PAGE 170)

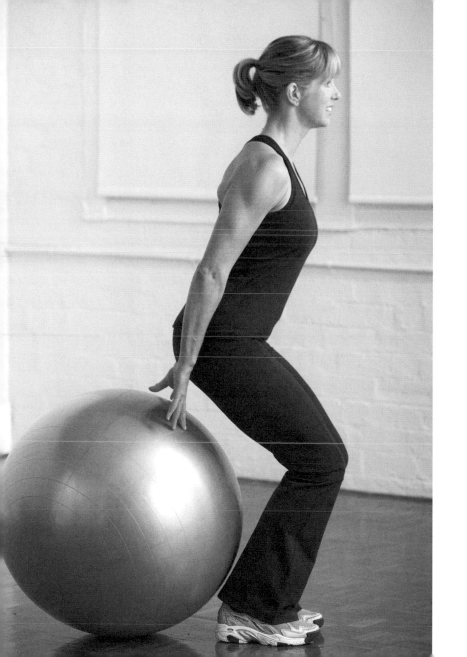

BANDS
AND BICEPS

bend and stretch for arm definition

Starting position

> Sit tall on the ball with your feet forward so you can see your toes beyond your knees.

> Place the center of the band under your feet.

> Hold each end of the band so that, with your arms straight and hands by your sides, the band is on slight tension.

> Make sure your elbows are tucked in close, your shoulders are relaxed and your core muscles are switched on.

Action

Bend and extend your elbows

> Bend you elbows, keeping them close to your sides, to stretch the band towards your shoulders

> Slowly straighten your elbows to release the tension smoothly.

> 15 x 2

Decrease the challenge

> Lengthen the band slightly or try a lighter band.

> Light weights are an alternative.

Increase the challenge

> Extend one knee to raise your foot off the floor.

> Slightly shorten the band for increased resistance.

Go harder

> Working one arm only, on the same side as the raised leg, will further challenge core control.

TRAINER TIPS

FOCUS ON A LONG STRONG SPINE AND KEEP YOUR CORE MUSCLES SWITCHED ON.

KEEP YOUR ELBOWS BY YOUR SIDE.

AVOID SHOULDER SHRUG.

LEVEL 3 HAND WEIGHTS CAN REPLACE THE BAND.

STRETCH

HIP AND CHEST STRETCH (SEE PAGE 170)

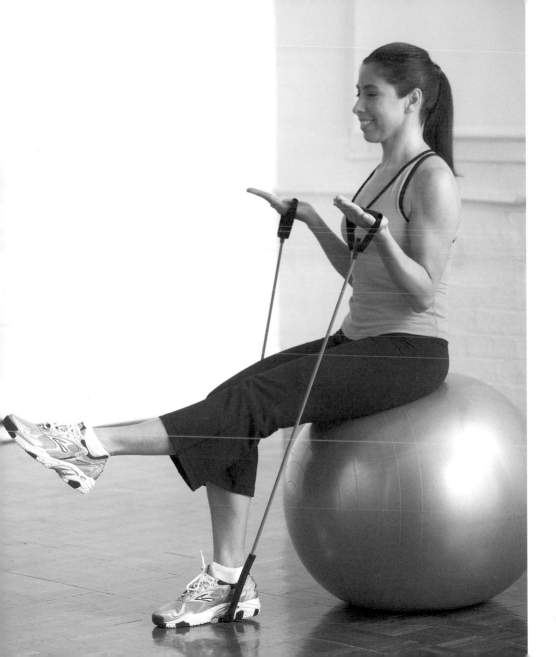

LATERAL ARM RAISE

shapely shoulders

Starting position
> Sit on the ball, feet hip-width apart, spine long and strong.
> Place the center of your band under your feet.
> With your elbows close to your sides, bend your forearms up to 90 degree angles, so they are parallel to the top of your thighs.
> Elongate your spine and set your core.

Action
Raise your arms sideways
> Draw your shoulder blades gently downwards.
> Raise your arms to shoulder height, palms facing downwards.
> 15 reps x 2 sets.

Decrease the challenge
> Lengthen the band or choose a band with less resistance.
> Use light weights or no load at all.

Increase the challenge
> Use a heavier band.
> Hold one leg raised for each set.

Go harder
> Perform a single arm lateral raise on the ball in combination with a leg extension to further test your core control. Working the arm on the same side as the raised leg is most challenging.

TRAINER TIPS

BE SURE YOUR SHOULDER BLADES STAY DOWN. AVOID SHRUGGING.

LEVEL 2 HAND WEIGHTS MAY BE USED INSTEAD OF THE BAND.

STRETCH

SHOULDER ROLLS (SEE PAGE 36)

NECK SEMI-CIRCLES (SEE PAGE 177)

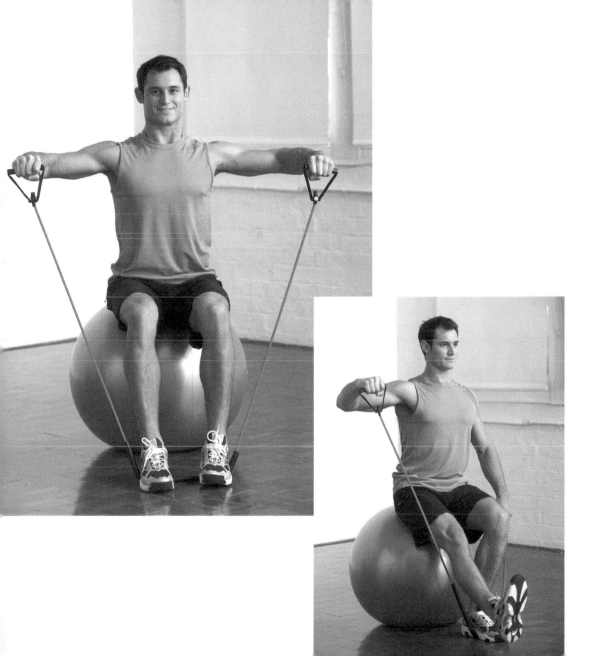

TRICEPS
WITH BAND

get those triceps toned and tough

Starting position
> Sit straight and strong on the ball with your feet hip width apart.
> Loop and tie, or shorten your band.
> Rest your stabilizing hand beside your shoulder with the elbow tucked in close to your side.
> Position your working arm beside your ear, the forearm over the top of your head.

Action
Extend one arm.
> Straighten the top arm, stretching the band towards the ceiling.
> Control it back down slowly.
> 15 reps on each side x 2

Decrease the challenge
> 10 each side
> Slightly lengthen the band or choose a lighter resistance.

Increase the challenge
> Place feet and knees together.
> Raise and lower your foot on the working arm side, straightening your knee as you stretch the band upwards.
> Increased resistance or reps.

TRAINER TIPS

KEEP BOTH ARMS TUCKED IN CLOSE BUT DO NOT LET YOUR TOP ARM CROSS YOUR FACE.

ALTERNATIVELY PERFORM A SINGLE ARM TRICEPS PRESS WITH A LEVEL ONE HAND WEIGHT.

STRETCH

SIDE STRETCH AND TRICEPS (SEE PAGE 174)

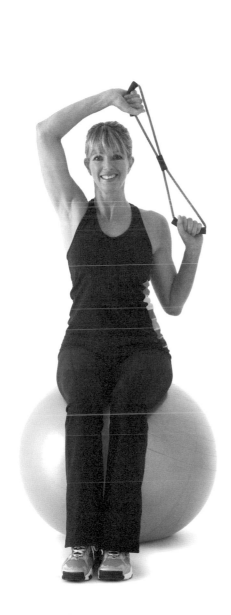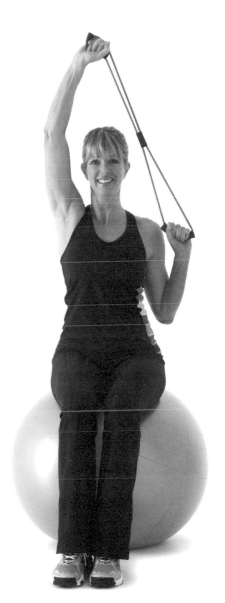

LAT
PULL DOWN
training for a beautiful back

Starting position
> Sit on the ball and engage your core muscles.
> Hold a shoulder-width portion of the band high above your head.
> Lengthen your neck and spine.
> Elbows are slightly bent and drawn gently back.

Action
Draw your hands down and out
> Retract your shoulder blades drawing them back and down.
> Continue the movement by bending your elbows downwards and outwards stretching your band as your hands arc outwards and down.
> Stop when the band is behind the top of your head.
> Slowly release the tension to return to the starting position.
> 15 reps x 2 sets

Unilateral control
> Hold the band still with one hand while the other arm performs the resisted lat pull down, bringing your elbow further down towards your hip.
> 12 reps on each side

Decrease the challenge
> Lighter resistance or fewer reps.

Increase the challenge
> Increased resistance or reps.
> Add alternating leg raise to the bilateral pull down.
> During the unilateral positions, hold your leg raised in front

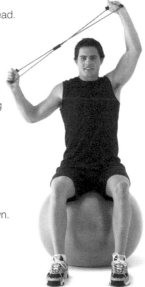

TRAINER TIPS

AVOID THE TEMPTATION TO LET YOUR SHOULDERS RIDE UP INTO A SHRUG POSITION BY FOCUSING ON DRAWING YOUR SHOULDER BLADES DOWN THROUGHOUT THE MOVEMENT.

STRETCH

BACK AND LATS STRETCH (SEE PAGE 165)

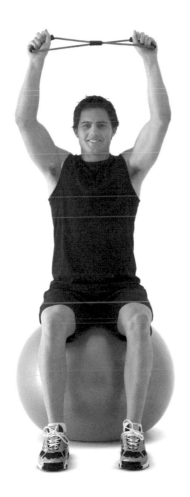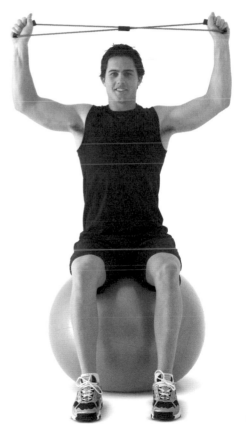

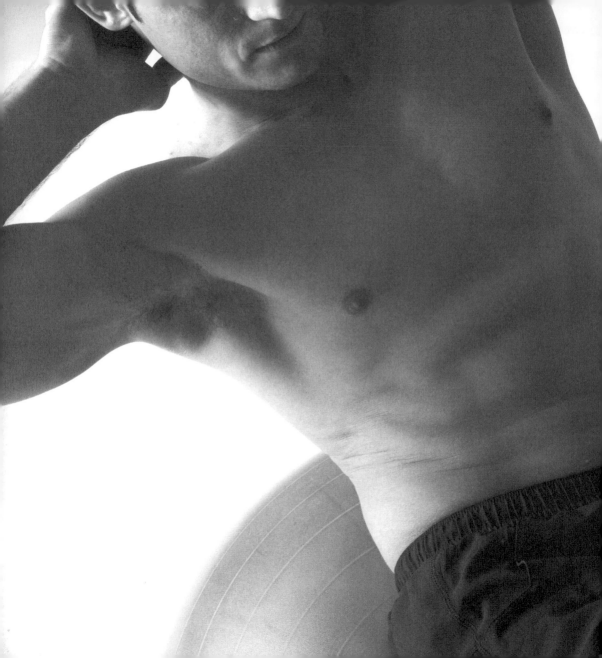

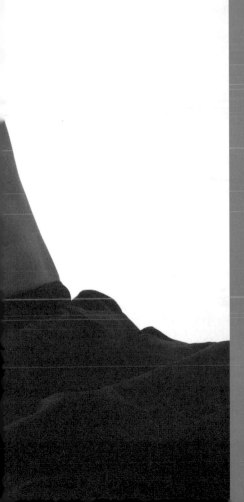

Train deep and outer abdominals together to give you a strong taut abdomen.

The following exercises provide variety and ab alternatives to regular ab curls on page 32.

If you have a back problem, ab curls are not for you. Instead, focus on core exercises such as those in the seated core section, until your back is pain free.

Revise your form

From the seated position, round your back, take a step forward and roll down slowly to lie back over the ball. Your tailbone must be touching the ball.

Place your hands under your head.

Gently draw your lower abdomen towards your lower back to engage your core.

Roll up and down one vertebra at a time, and curl up no further than halfway.

Keep your neck in line with your spine.

Two simple but effective ways to increase the challenges:

Bring your feet and knees together.

Take a small step back to roll a little further over the ball.

ALL ABOUT ABS

CURL
AND REACH

building on basic curls for your abs

Starting position
> Roll down to supine with the ball under your pelvis and lower back.
> Place your hands behind your head, elbows back, to support the weight of the head.

Action
Roll and reach

> Activate your deep abdominals by drawing them towards the ball.
> Reach one arm behind as you slowly curl up off the ball.
> Slowly roll back down, bringing your hand back behind your head.
> Repeat reaching out with the other arm.
> 16 reps x 2 sets

Decrease the challenge
> Take a small step forward, keeping your tailbone in contact with the ball.
> Perform the curl without the arm extension.

Increase the challenge
> Take a small step backwards.
> Bring your feet and knees together.
> 12 reps x 3 sets

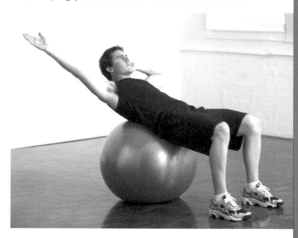

TRAINER TIPS

REST YOUR HEAD
IN YOUR HANDS.
AVOID PULLING WITH
YOUR ARMS.

KEEP YOUR NECK
IN LINE WITH SPINE,
CHIN OFF CHEST.

MAINTAIN DEEP
ABDOMINAL
ENGAGEMENT
THROUGHOUT
EVERY CURL.

STRETCH

SUPPORTED
CHEST STRETCH
(SEE PAGE 171)

STRETCH

HUG AND ARCH
(SEE PAGE 166)

CURL
AND EXTEND

balancing act for amazing abs

Action

Ab curl and leg raise

> Set your deep abdominals by drawing them towards the ball.

> Slowly curl your upper body up off the ball.

> Lift one foot off the floor, extending the knee.

> Replace your foot to the floor as you slowly roll back down.

> 12 reps x 2 sets

Decrease the challenge;

> Just raise your heel, leaving your toes on the floor.

Increase the challenge:

> Combine arm reach with opposite leg raise.

> 12 reps x 3 sets

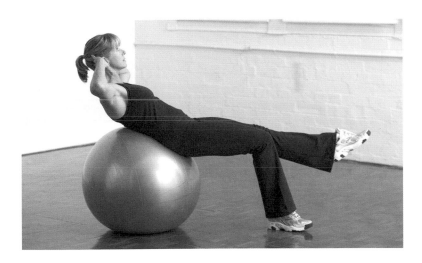

CURL
AND STEP

taking your ab curls one step further

Starting position
As for Curl and Extend on p101.

Action
Roll up and step back

> Draw your lower abdominals towards the ball.

> Slowly curl up maintaining a round back.

> Take a small step back with each foot.

> Step forward again.

> Roll back down.

Decrease the challenge
> Roll up and raise one heel then the other before rolling back down.

Increase the challenge
> Step slightly further back with each foot.

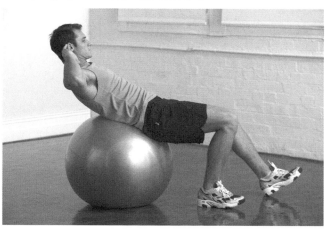

CURL SIDE REACH

hone in on your waist

Action
Curl up and reach sideways

> Draw your lower abdomen towards your lower back.

> Roll up and around to one side, reaching your hand past your knee to shorten that side of your body.

> Roll back slowly.

> 10 reps to each side x 2 sets

Decrease the challenge

> Lie on the floor and rest your legs on the ball. Reach up and around for your knee.

Increase the challenge

> Take a small step back with each foot.

> Bring your feet and knees together.

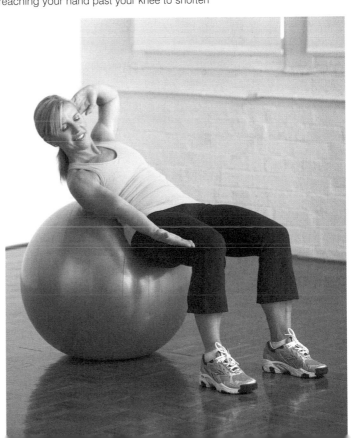

CLIMB
THE ROPE

strengthen your obliques

Starting position
> Supine on the ball, with your tailbone in contact with the ball.
> Arms reaching up to hold an imaginary rope that is hanging down above your chest.

Action
Reach one hand then the other as you roll up
> Climb your hands up the rope, step by step, raising one shoulder then the other.
> Slide back down the rope slowly.
> 15 reps x 2 sets

Decrease the challenge
> Lie on the floor with your legs relaxed on the ball.

Increase the challenge
> Bring your feet and knees together.

Go harder
> Roll over slightly onto one side on the ball.
> Reach your top arm for the imaginary rope.
> Your bottom hand supports your head, elbow pointing toward the floor.
> Raise and lower your arm and side of body slowly.
> x 15 each side

TRAINER TIPS

KEEP IT SLOW AND CONTROLLED.

STRETCH

ROTATION AND CHEST STRETCH (SEE PAGE 163)

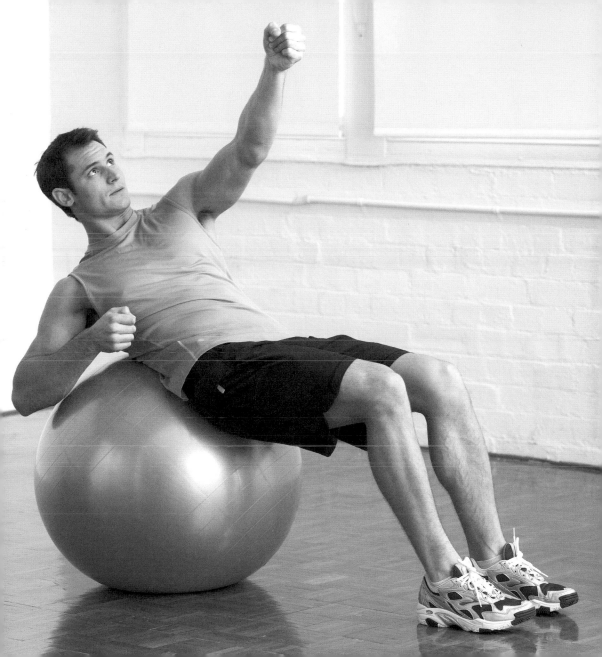

OVERHEAD CONTROL

a gentle exercise honing in on alignment

Starting position:

> Lie on the floor with your knees bent.
> Rest the ball on your abdomen.

Action

Keep your back still as you raise the ball overhead

> Draw your shoulders gently down away from your ears and draw your lower abdomen towards the floor.
> Focus on maintaining the neutral position of your spine.
> Slowly raise the ball up and over your head to the floor and back again.
> Do not allow your ribs to lift upward or your lower back to arch.

Decrease the challenge

> Perform this move without the ball.

Increase the challenge

> Perform the move with your legs straight on the floor.

TRAINER TIPS

BE AWARE OF THE NATURAL POSITION OF YOUR SPINE AND RIB CAGE BEFORE YOU MOVE THE BALL AND AIM TO MAINTAIN THIS AS THE BALL GOES OVERHEAD.

KEEP YOUR NECK AND SHOULDERS RELAXED.

STRETCH

ROTATION AND CHEST STRETCH
(SEE PAGE 163)

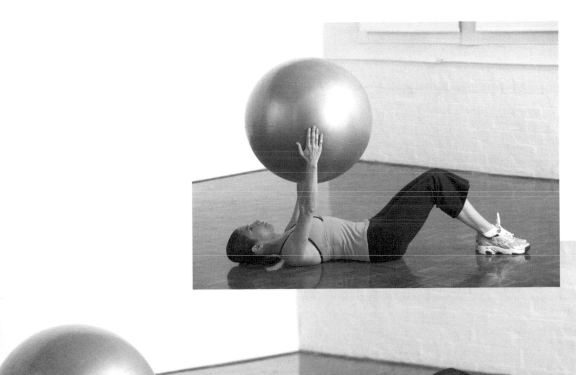

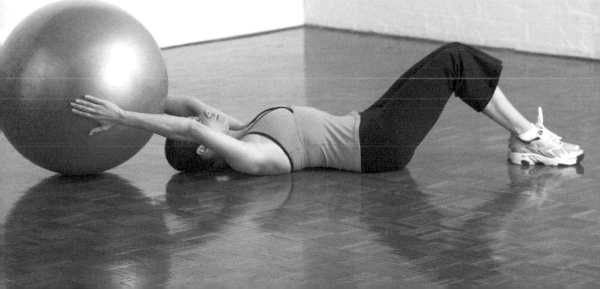

KNEE ROLL

slowly roll for smooth control

Starting position
> Lie supine on the floor, with your knees bent at 45 degrees, feet away from hips, holding ball resting on your abdomen.

Action

Roll the ball to your knees

> Draw your lower abdomen towards the floor to set your core.

> Slowly lift your head and shoulders and continue to curl up, as you roll the ball up your thighs to your knees.

> Roll back down with control.

> 15 reps x 3

Decrease the challenge
> Roll the ball just a little up your legs, lifting only head and shoulders.

Increase the challenge
> To focus on obliques, roll the ball up and over to one knee turning your upper body slightly. Add 15 to each side to your straight knee rolls.

TRAINER TIPS

KEEP YOUR DEEP ABDOMINALS ENGAGED AND CURL YOUR SPINE ONE VERTEBRA AT A TIME.

STRETCH

HUG AND ARCH OR HIP AND CHEST STRETCH (SEE PAGE 166)

OR HIP AND CHEST STRETCH (SEE PAGE 170)

OR ROTATION AND CHEST STRETCH (SEE PAGE 163)

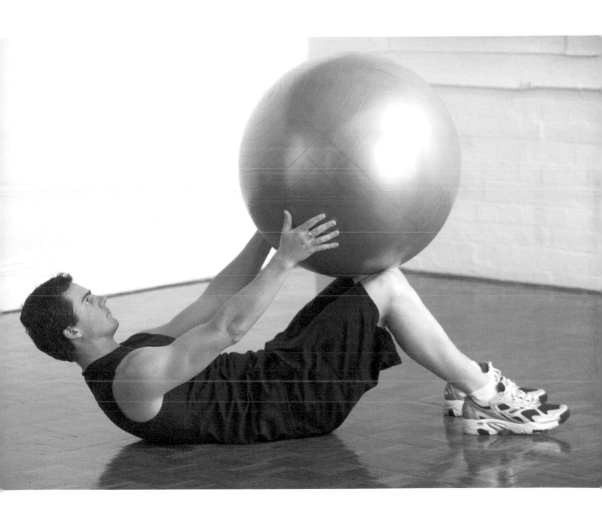

ROLL
AWAY V

V for variety to the original roll away

Starting position

> Upright kneeling, with your arms outstretched to the ball in front, fingers resting on the ball.

> Settle your shoulders back and down, engage your deep abdominals and lightly switch on your gluteals to be sure you keep your hips straight.

Action

Lean forward and stay stable as you roll the ball

> Roll the ball away as you incline forward.

> Roll off your knees to rest on your thighs on the floor and your forearms on the ball.

> Keep the straight alignment from your ears to your knees.

> Be sure your shoulders are drawing downwards and deep abdominals are switched on to support your spine.

> Holding your body stable, slowly roll the ball forward to one side, back to the center and then forward to the second side.

> Continue to angle the ball away and back, side to side.

> 5 rolls each side.

Decrease the challenge

> Perform the original roll away without the V.

> Try the wall hover on page 82.

Increase the challenge

> Roll the ball further forward on each side.

TRAINER TIPS

BE SURE TO GET OFF YOUR KNEES BY BRINGING YOUR FEET UP TOWARDS YOUR HIPS.

DON'T LET YOUR UPPER BACK ROUND OR YOUR LOWER BACK SWAY.

BREATHE EVENLY.

STRETCH

BACK AND LATS STRETCH (SEE PAGE 165)

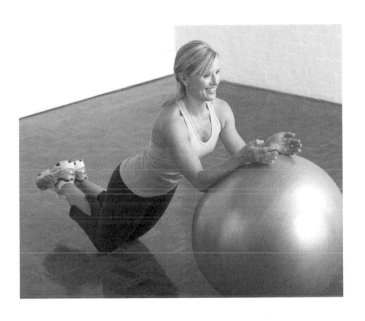

BALL
HOVER

an advanced abdominal challenge for those
comfortable and confident on the ball

Starting position

> Kneel on the floor with your forearms resting on the ball
  and toes tucked under.

> Set your shoulders downwards, and draw your lower abdomen
  towards your lower back.

Action

Lift and hold straight and strong

> Raise your knees and lift into a position of straight alignment top to toe.

> Hold this position, keeping your shoulders down, upper back straight
  and lower back supported and stable in the neutral position.

> Hold for 5 slow breaths, repeat x 4.

Decrease the challenge

> Lift your knees just a little off the floor, hold for 3 breaths and lower.

> Do the wall hover on p82.

Increase the challenge

> Hover run: Bend one knee then the other towards the floor keeping
  your lower back and
  pelvis absolutely still.

Go harder

> Raise one foot off the
  floor keeping the leg
  straight.

> Hold for 3 breaths.

> x 3 on each leg

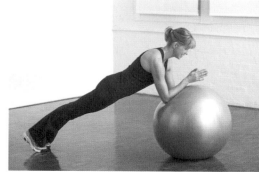

TRAINER TIPS

KEEP YOUR CHEST UP.
DON'T LET IT DROOP
OVER THE BALL.

STRAIGHT ALIGNMENT
IS ESSENTIAL.

STRETCH

HUG AND ARCH
(SEE PAGE 166)

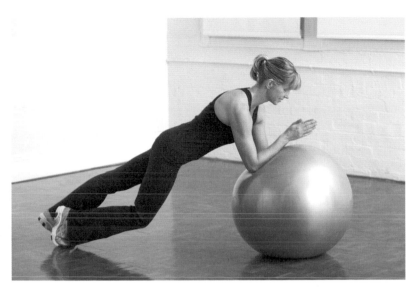

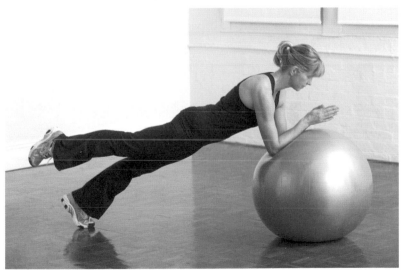

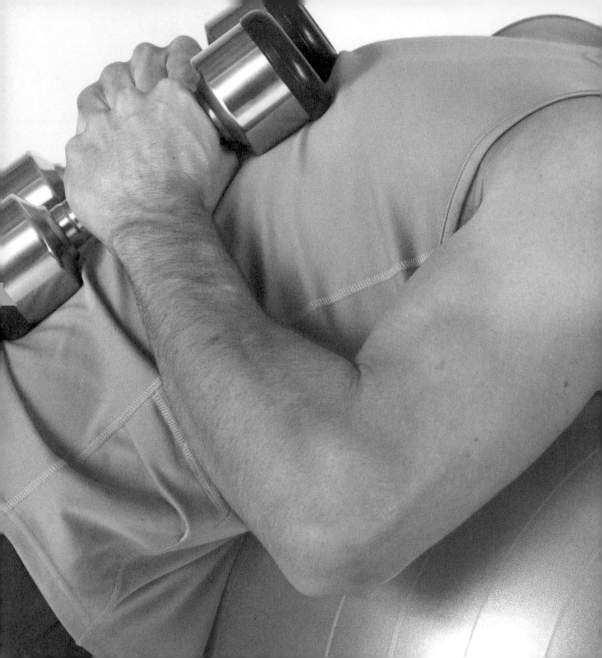

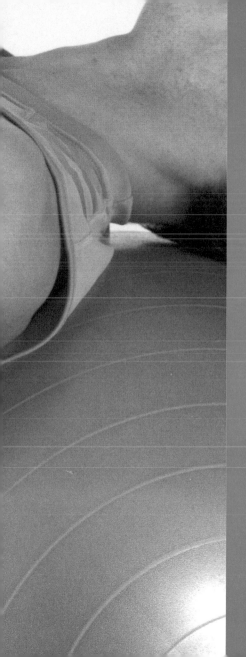

Work your back, butt, core and more

Originally, lying face up on the ball was used to add challenge to traditional exercises such as chest press and flys (page 31). On the ball, more muscles are used, particularly in your back and butt and there is added training of stability and balance.

The following exercises provide new alternatives for training in this position, with equal or more emphasis on gluteals, back strength and stability.

To get there:

Sit with your hands resting on the ball.

Round your back. Walk your feet forward and roll your body down to rest your elbows on the ball.

Continue to walk your feet out until your shoulder blades are on the ball.

Now lay your head back and lift your hips to establish the strong "table-like" supine on the ball position.

Your heels should be directly under your knees and hip-width apart initially. (Closer together is more challenging.)

Be sure that your head, neck and shoulders are well supported by the ball and your neck is in line with your spine.

If your chin is on your chest, roll back a little and if your head is hanging back, walk further forward.

SUPINE ON THE BALL

SUPINE ROTATION

strong back, great butt

Starting position

> Supine on the ball with your head, neck and shoulders on the ball and your bottom raised so your body and thighs are in line and horizontal.

> Press through your heels to keep your hips raised.

> Draw your lower abdomen towards your lower back to support your lumbar spine.

> Hold a level 3 hand weight in both hands, arms extended towards the ceiling.

Action

Slowly rotate the weight

> Slowly rotate from side to side, taking the weight in a wide arc around your upper body. The ball and your upper body will roll.

> Keep your hips upright and level.

Decrease the challenge

> Perform this without a weight.

Increase the challenge

> Keep your feet and knees together.

TRAINER TIPS

CONTINUE TO ENGAGE YOUR DEEP ABDOMINALS TO SUPPORT YOUR LOWER BACK.

STRETCH

SEATED HAMSTRING STRETCH (SEE PAGE 172)

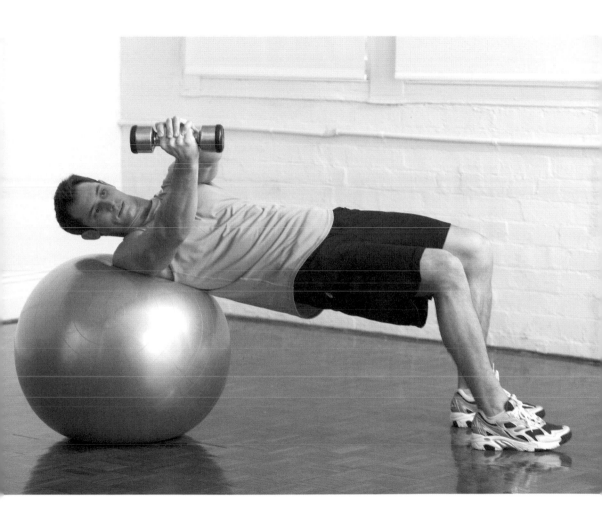

SUPINE
PEC PASS

perfect pecs plus postural precision

Starting position
> Roll down to supine on the ball, head to shoulder blades supported.
> Neck in line with spine.
> Hips held raised, legs and body in a horizontal line.
> Be sure your feet are hip-width apart and your heels are under your knees.
> Hold one level 2 hand weight above your chest, your elbows slightly bent.
> Engage your deep abs and push through your heels as you switch on your gluteals.

Action
Pass the weight, control the ball
> Slowly perform a one-hand fly lowering the weight down and sideways until your arm is level with your shoulder.
> Arc the weight back up, change hands above your chest and then lower the weight outward to the second side.
> Continue to pass the weight from hand to hand, focusing on keeping your ball and body still and stable.
> 10 reps each side

Decrease the challenge
> Level 1 or no weight
> 5 reps on each side

Increase the challenge
> Level 3 weight
> Feet and knees together

TRAINER TIP

KEEP YOUR ELBOWS SLIGHTLY BENT.

USE YOUR GLUTEALS TO KEEP YOUR HIPS RAISED AND YOUR DEEP ABDOMINALS TO SUPPORT YOUR SPINE.

STRETCH

ROTATION AND CHEST STRETCH (SEE PAGE 163)

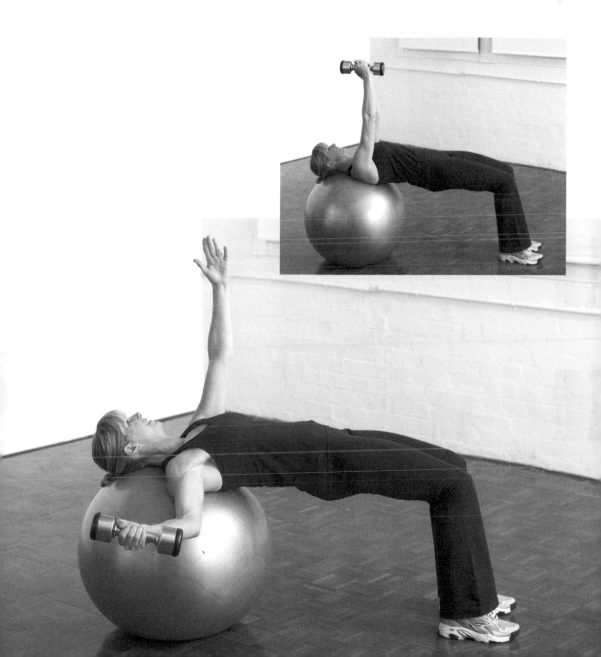

SUPINE GLIDE

blitz your back and butt

Starting position
> Lie supine on the ball.
> Feet hip-width apart, heels under knees.
> Lower your hips towards the floor.
> Rest your hands under your head.

Action
Raise, and roll

> Set your core.
> Push through your heels and use your gluteals to raise your hips to horizontal.
> Roll the ball backwards, straightening your knees. Keep your hips held high.
> Roll forward to return to bent knees.
> Relax your hips back down.
> 15 reps x 2

Decrease the challenge
> Raise and lower your hips slowly but do not roll back.

Increase the challenge:
> Knees and feet closer together.

Go harder
> Shift your weight into one foot, using the other foot lightly on the floor for balance only.
> Keep your hips in line as you roll back bearing your weight through one leg.
> 10 on each side.

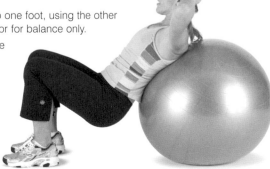

TRAINER TIPS

FOCUS ON SLOW CONTROLLED MOVEMENTS.

KEEP YOUR DEEP ABS ENGAGED TO SUPPORT YOUR BACK.

STRETCH

SEATED HAMSTRING STRETCH (SEE PAGE 172)

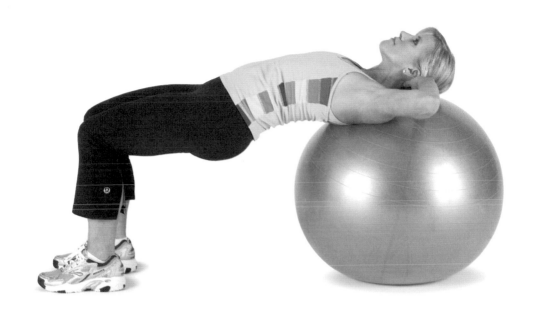

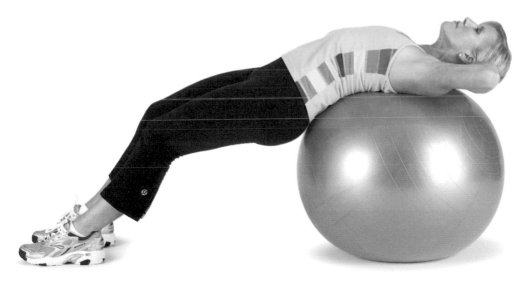

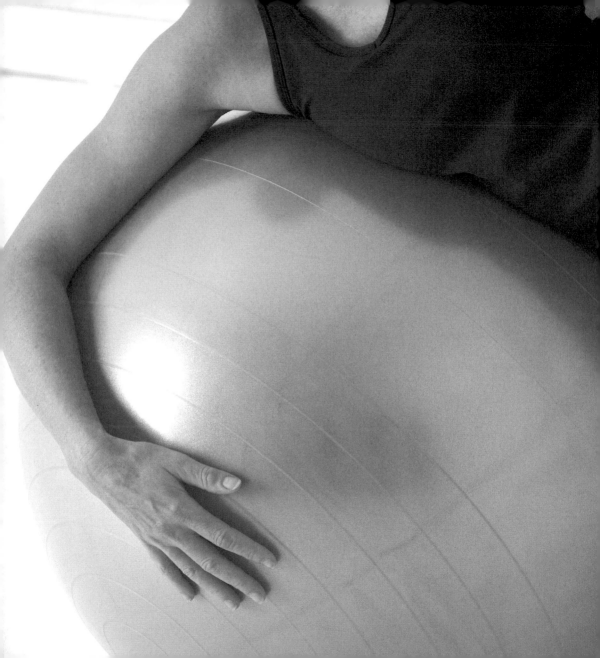

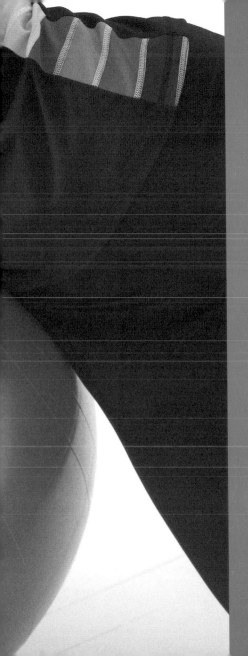

Lying sideways over the ball or hovered side-on puts extra focus on your lateral muscles.

Because of the forward and back movement the first exercise requires more core control than the original side leg raise, while the side lean variation includes extra thigh focus compared with the original side lean.

Thigh and waist conditioning are a major emphasis in the next two exercises. Shoulder stability and lateral trunk control are also required.

SIDE-ON

LEG RAISE
FORWARD AND BACK
control the roll

Adding forward and backward movement to this popular thigh strengthening exercise adds a whole new meaning to core control.

Starting position

> Start off kneeling upright with the ball firmly against your thigh.
> Lie sideways over the ball and extend your outside leg.
> Slide your supporting knee a little outward to find a comfortable position.
> Elongate your body over the ball.
> Support your head in your hand and engage your deep abdominals.

Action

Raise and lower your leg forward and back

> Raise your leg to hip height.
> Keep your leg long and strong as you lower your foot forward to touch the floor in front.
> Raise your leg back to horizontal and in line with your body.
> Now lower it downward and backward to touch the floor behind.
> Use your core control to keep your pelvis and the ball still while your leg moves forward and back.
> 15 reps x 2 sets each leg

Decrease the challenge

> Raise your leg directly up and down.
> Lie on your side on the floor.

Increase the challenge

> Add leg circles after 15 reps. Hold your leg straight and strong and perform 5 slow circles in each direction.

TRAINER TIPS

FOCUS ON KEEPING YOUR BODY LONG AND THE BALL STABLE.

KEEP YOUR KNEE AND FOOT FACING FORWARD, AVOID TURNING THEM UPWARDS.

STRETCH

BACK AND LATS STRETCH (SEE PAGE 165)

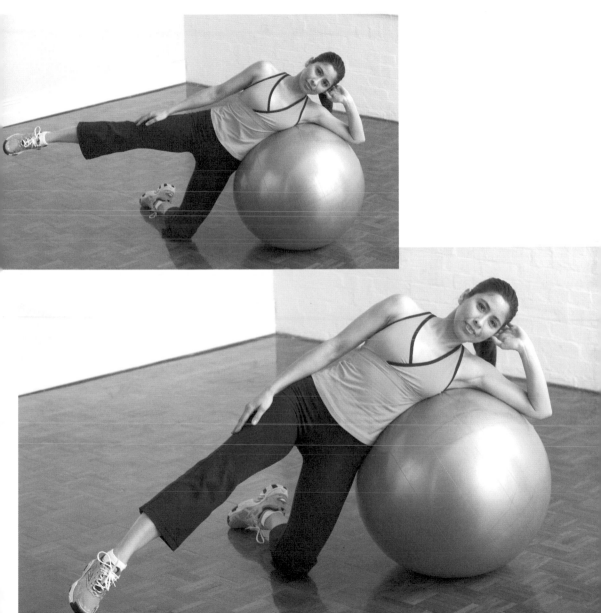

SIDE LEAN AND RAISE

lateral control with added butt bonus

Starting position
> Kneel upright with the ball beside you but it should not touch your leg.
> Rest the side of your hand on the ball keeping your elbows close to your body.
> Set your postural alignment; shoulders back and down, abdominals drawn in gently.

Action
Lean sideways and add lateral leg lift

> Tilt sideways to lean through your forearm on the ball, keeping your body in a straight line.
> Hold the side lean as you slowly raise and lower your leg x 10.
> 2 sets each side

Decrease the challenge
Perform the side lean without the leg lift.

Increase the challenge
> 15 reps each leg x 2 sets
> Hold a weight resting against your outer thigh as close to your knee as possible.

TRAINER TIPS

KEEP YOUR SHOULDERS DRAWN BACK AND DOWN. DO NOT LET YOUR SUPPORTING SHOULDER ROLL FORWARD.

AVOID BENDING SIDEWAYS. YOU SHOULD MAINTAIN A STRAIGHT LINE FROM YOUR NOSE THROUGH YOUR NAVEL TO THE POINT WHERE YOUR KNEES MEET IN THE MIDDLE.

OBSERVE YOUR FORM IN THE MIRROR.

STRETCH

KNEELING SIDE STRETCH (SEE PAGE 168)

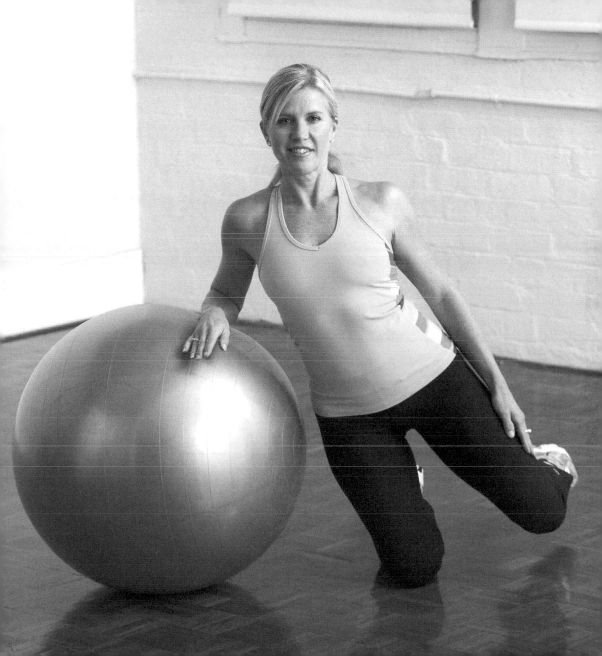

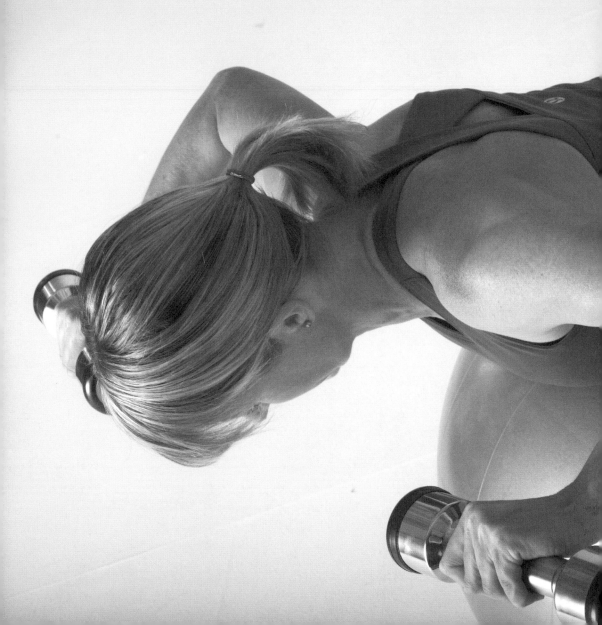

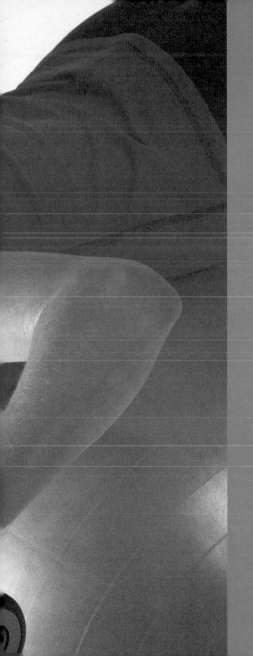

Lie prone to help you stand tall

Lying prone over the ball allows you to strengthen the important posterior muscle groups. These groups are too often neglected in other training programs because they are "out of sight, out of mind," but are vital for a balanced body. Working your back and butt muscles gives you fabulous posture, a strong back and core.

By lying prone on the ball, you back is well supported and your body is up off the floor enabling you to train your back, butt, shoulders and thighs safely and effectively.

The following exercises are variations for tried and true prone options such as arm raise or leg raise (page 32).

PRONE ON THE BALL

BREASTSTROKE

swim your way to a strong stunning back

Starting position
> Prone on the ball.
> Feet hip-width apart on the floor. Push your heels back so your are leaning through the balls of your feet.
> Hold your chest up to enhance back strength and alignment.
> Rest your hands lightly on the ball.
> Look at the floor to keep your neck in line with your spine.

Action
Reach your arms forward and around
> Settle your shoulder blades back and down to open across your chest.
> Reach your arms forward in the midline, then arc them out and around to your hips. Continue this slow breaststroke action bringing your hands together in front of your chest ready to "swim" again.
> Rest back off the ball, kneeling on the floor between sets.
> 15 x 2 sets

Decrease the challenge
> Perform single arm breaststroke leaving your other hand resting lightly on the floor.

Increase the challenge
> Add alternating straight leg raise to bring your butt into the picture, further challenging strength and control.

TRAINER TIPS

HOLD YOUR CHEST UP
OFF THE BALL AND
KEEP YOUR NECK IN
LINE WITH YOUR SPINE.

STRETCH

BACK AND
LATS STRETCH
(SEE PAGE 165)

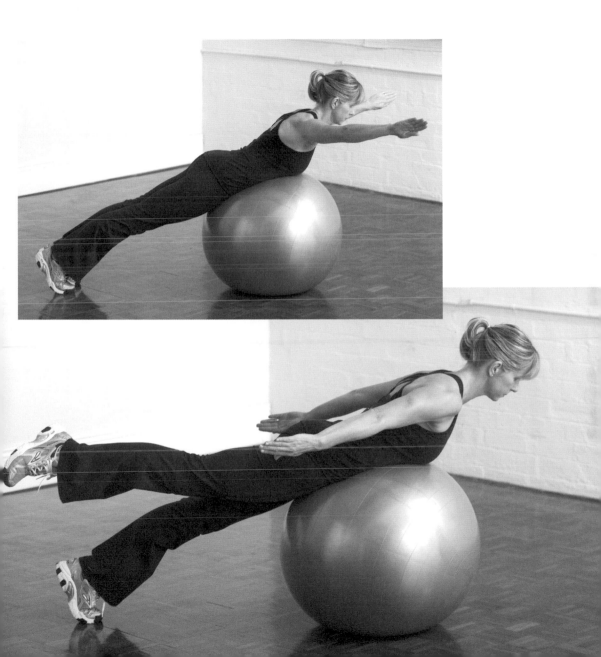

KNEELING EXTENSION

focus on upper back to build perfect posture

Starting position
> Kneeling upright, place the ball firmly against your thighs.
> Lengthen your spine as you wrap your body over the ball, molding to it's shape.
> Rest your hands on the ball in front of your body.
> Walk your knees in under the ball.

Action
Raise your chest and shoulders, extend your upper body off the ball
> Keep your abdomen and legs in contact with the ball.
> Draw your shoulders back and down towards your tailbone to open across your chest.
> Continue by raising your head and chest slowly to "peel" up off the ball.
> Simultaneously reach your arm forward, turning your palm up and out.
> Roll back down to the round relaxed position replacing your hand on the ball.
> Repeat raising your other arm.
> 12 reps (6 each arm) x 2 sets

Decrease the challenge
> Leave your hands on the ball to provide light support as you gently extend your upper back. 5 x 2 sets (rest back off the ball in between sets).

Increase the challenge
> Reach both arms together up and out as you raise your chest and peel off the ball.

TRAINER TIPS

KEEP YOUR BODY LONG OVER THE BALL.

SLOW CONTROL IS ESSENTIAL.

TO ISOLATE AND STRENGTHEN YOUR UPPER BACK, KEEP YOUR ABDOMEN ON THE BALL.

STRETCH

UPPER BACK STRETCH (SEE PAGE 175)

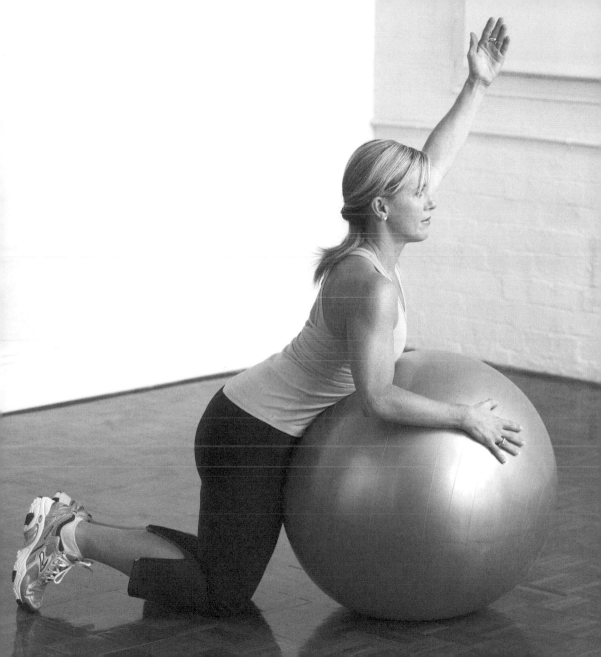

PRONE ROW
WITH BAND

upper back focus for fantastic posture

Starting position

> Prone over the ball, feet hip width apart or closer, weight bearing into the balls of your feet by pushing your heels backwards.

> Hold a resistance band between your hands on the floor, shoulder-width apart.

> Raise your chest slightly to engage your back muscles.

> Look at the floor in front of your band to maintain healthy neck alignment.

Action

Draw your arms out wide

> Engage the muscles to set your shoulder blades down towards your tailbone.

> Draw your shoulder blades inwards to start the movement.

> Bend and raise your elbows outwards to take your hands up and wide.

> The band will travel upwards, just in front of the ball as it stretches.

> Slowly release the band back to the floor.

> 15 reps x 2 sets.

Decrease the challenge

> This exercise can be performed sitting on the ball, holding the band in front of your chest.

> Use a lighter band or no band to lighten the load.

> 5 reps x 3

Increase the challenge

> Increase the band resistance or hold it a little shorter.

> Increase reps or sets.

> Add alternating single leg raise.

TRAINER TIPS

LEVEL 1 HAND WEIGHTS CAN BE USED INSTEAD OF THE BAND.

FOCUS ON USING THE MUSCLES BETWEEN YOUR SHOULDER BLADES, KEEPING THEM DOWN AS THEY DRAW TOGETHER.

MONITOR YOUR FORM FOR QUALITY FLOWING MOVEMENT.

STRETCH

UPPER BACK STRETCH (SEE PAGE 175)

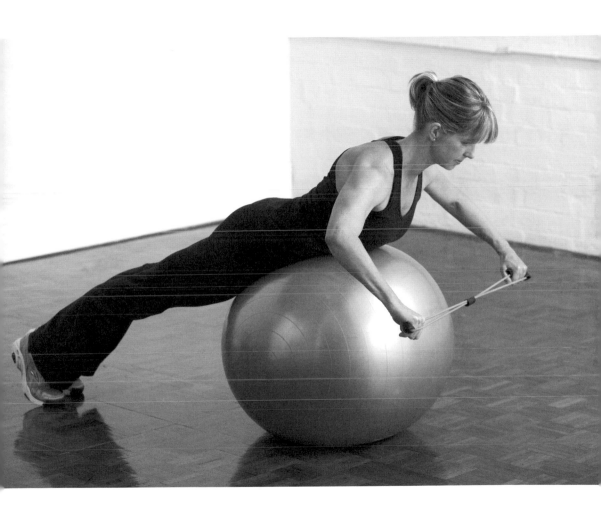

PRONE TRICEPS WITH BAND

strong arms and back

Starting position

> Lie prone on the ball with your feet firmly on the floor.

> Slide the middle of the band firmly under the front of the ball.

> Holding the band ends, bend your elbows up and tuck your arms in, close by your sides.

> Draw your shoulders down and have your chest raised slightly to activate your back muscles.

> Look at the floor to avoid straining your neck.

Action

Straighten your elbows to stretch the band

> Keep your upper arms held high and still.

> Extend your elbows back stretching the band as you straighten your elbows.

> Keep your shoulder blades away from your ears.

> Release slowly.

> 15 x 2 sets

Decrease the challenge

> 10 x 2 sets

> Slightly lengthen the band.

> Perform the move without resistance.

Increase the challenge

> Slightly shorten the band or select a heavier resistance.

> Increase the reps or sets.

> Add alternate straight leg raise, lifting your foot hip height as you push back.

TRAINER TIPS

KEEP YOUR NECK IN LINE WITH YOUR SPINE.

HOLD YOUR ELBOWS HIGHER THAN YOUR MIDDLE BACK AND KEEP THEM TUCKED IN.

DO NOT ROLL THE BALL BACK OFF THE BAND.

LEVEL 2 HAND WEIGHTS CAN BE USED INSTEAD OF THE RESISTANCE BAND.

STRETCH

SIDE STRETCH AND TRICEPS (SEE PAGE 174)

BACK AND LATS STRETCH (SEE PAGE 165)

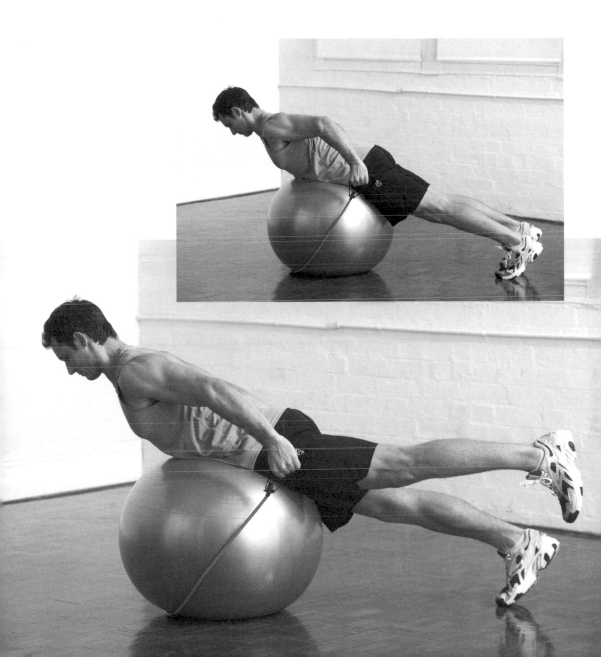

SCISSORS

butt buster

Starting position

> Lie prone on the ball, legs horizontal and extended.
> Raise your chest slightly, so your fingers are resting lightly on the floor.
> Keep your neck in line with your spine.

Action

Criss-cross your legs keeping them very straight and strong

> Keep your legs straight and horizontal, as you take them outward then bring them back to cross one over the other in the midline.
> Alternate which leg crosses on top.
> 16 x 2 sets

Decrease the challenge

> Decrease reps and sets.
> Perform single leg raise resting your other foot on the ground.
> x 10 each side.

Increase the challenge

> Add single arm reach to each.

Go harder

> To truly test your balance, try both arms raised. Try to balance with your legs horizontal but still initially.
> Once you have achieved this add the leg scissors continuing to focus on good form.

TRAINER TIPS

KEEP YOUR SHOULDERS AND FEET HIP HEIGHT AND YOUR NECK IN LINE WITH YOUR SPINE.

FOCUSING ON LONG, STRONG, STRAIGHT LEGS WILL OPTIMIZE YOUR BUTT WORKOUT.

STRETCH

CIRCLE AND HUG
(SEE PAGE 162)

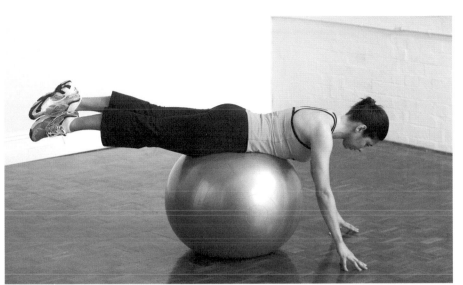

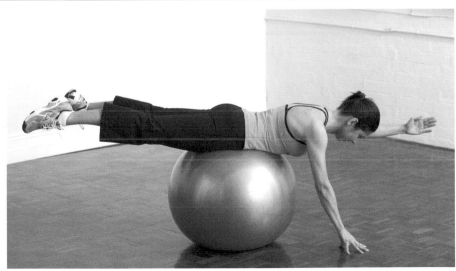

CROSSED LEG EXTENSION

the pièce de résistance of butt busters

Starting position
> Set up your balanced prone position, body and legs straight, strong and horizontal.
> Fingers are resting lightly on the floor.
> Cross one leg over the other.

Action

Lift with your lower leg as you resist with the top one.
> Keep your legs straight and tightly crossed and your chest up off the ball.
> Lower your legs halfway towards the floor.
> Push down with the top leg as you lift with the bottom leg to bring them back to horizontal height.
> 15 reps x 2 sets on each leg, resting back off the ball between each set.

Decrease the challenge
> Single leg raise and lower, with your other foot leaning on the floor x 10 each side.

Increase the challenge
> Extend and hold your opposite arm forward at shoulder height.

Go harder
> To truly train back strength balance and control progress to holding both arms off the floor.

TRAINER TIPS

THE MORE YOU RESIST THE MOVEMENT WITH YOUR TOP LEG, THE HARDER YOUR BOTTOM LEG WILL WORK.

STAY LIGHT ON YOUR FINGERTIPS: THE LESS YOU LEAN ON YOUR HANDS THE MORE YOU STRENGTHEN YOUR BACK AND BALANCE.

STRETCH

BACK AND LATS STRETCH (SEE PAGE 165)

POSTERIOR HIP STRETCH (SEE PAGE 173)

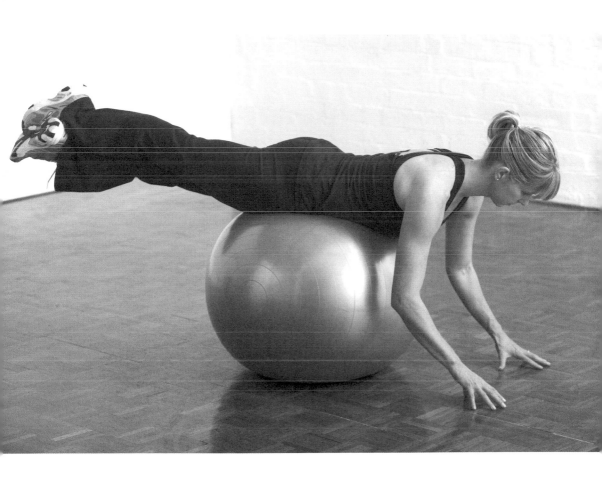

DIAMOND
LEG LIFT

hamstrings, gluteals and backs unite

Starting position
> Lie prone on the ball, your legs straight and together.
> Chest raised slightly and fingers resting lightly on the floor for balance.
> Look at the floor.

Action
Bend, lift, lower and straighten legs.
> Keep your feet together at all times.
> Bend your knees to 90 degrees, taking them wide but keep your feet touching (this creates a diamond shape).
> Use your gluteals to lift both legs just a little. Keep your upper body still.
> Lower your knees back to hip height.
> Squeeze your legs straight and together.
> 15 x 2 sets

Decrease the challenge
> Leave one foot on the floor, raise and lower the other leg, keeping it straight and strong.
> Hold the other leg at hip height and bend it and straighten it x 10.
> Rest back off the ball then repeat on the second leg.

Increase the challenge
> Perform a third set.

TRAINER TIPS

AVOID THE TEMPTATION TO LOWER YOUR CHEST AS YOUR LEGS PUSH UPWARDS.

REALLY SQUEEZE YOUR LEGS STRAIGHT AND TOGETHER.

STRETCH

CIRCLE AND HUG (SEE PAGE 162)

BACK AND LATS STRETCH (SEE PAGE 165)

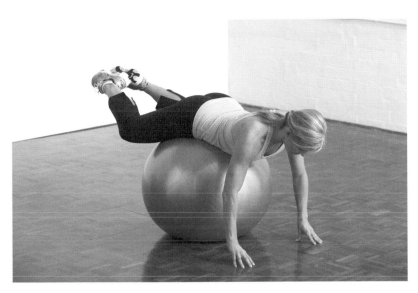

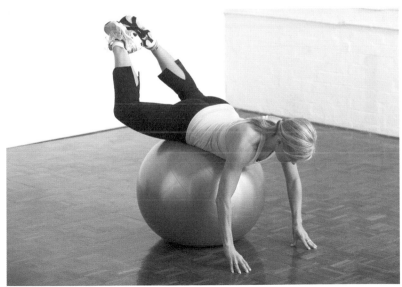

143

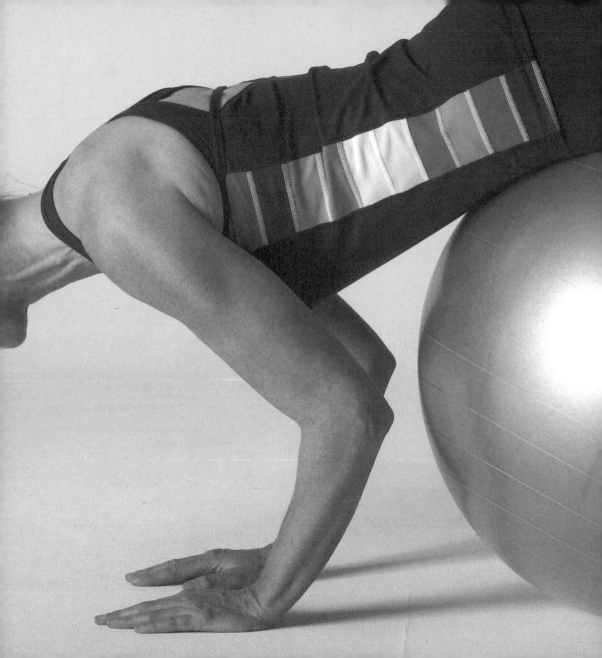

Traditionally used for push-ups, the forward prone position works shoulders, abs, core and more.

The moment you roll forward from the horizontal prone position and your abdomen and back are no longer supported you are in the forward prone position. This means you are taking at least some weight through your hands and you need shoulder and spinal stability to control your posture and the ball.

A popular and common exercise in this position is the ball push-up (p33) but simply walking out to the push-up position is a fabulous way to train strength and stability as you will discover with the prone walkout. For those looking for a new angle to the original ball push-up, there's the uneven push-up and the triceps alternative too.

If you are used to performing push-ups easily on the floor, take care, the ball adds significant core challenge. The further you walk out over the ball, the tougher the workout. Be sure to maintain perfect alignment before you take that extra step forward.

FORWARD PRONE

PRONE
WALK OUT

slowly and surely strengthen your shoulders and spine

Starting position
> Lie over the ball balanced in the prone position.
> Your abdomen is on the ball, and your legs elevated to be straight and in line with your body.
> Fingers resting lightly on the floor, neck in line with spine.

Action
Slowly and purposely walk out

> Settle your shoulders towards your tailbone and engage your deep abdominals.
> Very slowly, as though in slow motion, walk out over the ball.
> Lift each hand high and place it carefully on the floor as though you are a lion in the jungle stalking your prey.
> Focus on keeping your shoulders and back in perfect alignment.
> Keep your back straight and strong.
> Take 2 steps forward with each hand, then slowly reverse the movement until you are back balanced on the ball with fingertips resting lightly on the floor (with no weight through your hands).
> Repeat x 5

Decrease the challenge
> Roll slightly forward to take just a small amount of weight through your hands. Slowly glide your weight from one hand to the other by rolling the ball carefully side to side.
> Alternatively walk out just one step with each hand.

Increase the challenge
> Walk out 3 steps on each hand.

TRAINER TIPS

THE MOMENT YOUR ABDOMEN ROLLS FORWARD YOU MUST ACTIVATE YOUR DEEP ABDOMINALS TO SUPPORT YOUR SPINE.

DON'T LET YOUR BACK ARCH OR YOUR PELVIS ROCK OR DROP FROM SIDE TO SIDE. VISUALIZE A GLASS OF WATER BALANCED ON YOUR LOWER BACK. DON'T LET IT SPILL.

REMEMBER QUALITY NOT QUANTITY.

STRETCH

BACK AND LATS STRETCH (SEE PAGE 165)

NECK SEMI-CIRCLES (SEE PAGE 177)

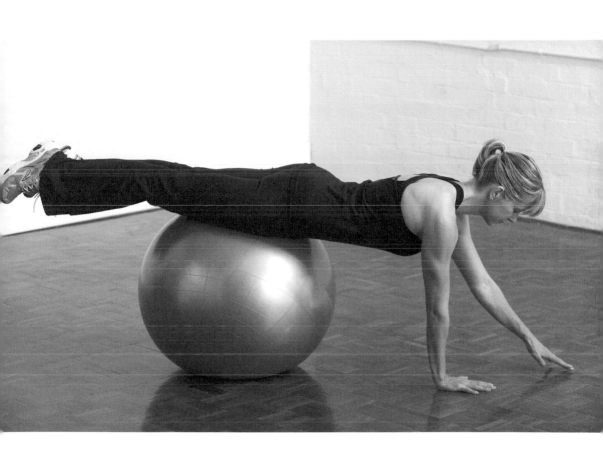

UNEVEN PUSH-UP

a fresh approach to an old favorite

Starting position

> Prone and balanced on the ball with legs extended.
> Engage shoulder and spinal stabilizers.
> Walk your hands out one or two steps as though ready to perform a push-up.
> Take an extra step forward with one hand.
> Roll slightly more weight into the hand that is behind.

Action

Slowly press down and up

> Bend your elbows to lower your chest towards the floor.
> Slowly press back up.
> 10 reps then switch arm position.

Decrease the challenge

> Try the regular ball push-up (page 33).
> Perform the uneven push-up with the ball under your hips. Gradually walk your hands out further as you develop strength and control.

Increase the challenge

> Walk further out over the ball.
> To hone in on single arm strength, roll your body weight further onto the back hand so the front hand is for balance only.

TRAINER TIPS

AVOID LOCKING YOUR ELBOWS.

DO NOT LET YOUR BACK SWAY.

FOCUS ON KEEPING YOUR SHOULDER BLADES DRAWN AWAY FROM YOUR EARS.

STRETCH

HIP AND CHEST STRETCH (SEE PAGE 170)

SUPPORTED CHEST STRETCH (SEE PAGE 171)

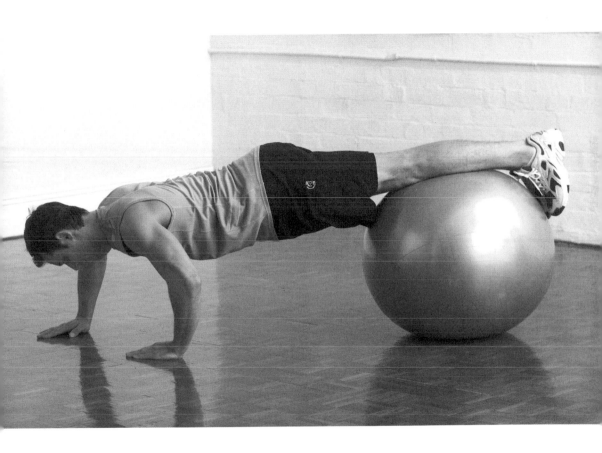

TRICEPS
PUSH-UP

put your triceps to the test

Starting position
> Lie in the prone horizontal position, straight and strong on the ball with legs elevated and together.
> Neck in line with spine.
> Set your shoulder blades and activate your core abdominals.
> Walk out 2 steps with each hand.
> Place the heels of your hands directly under your shoulders, with your fingers pointing forwards.

Action
Bend your elbows towards the ball to lower your chest
> Slowly bend your elbows down and towards the ball to lower your chest towards the floor.
> Press back up.
> 12 reps x 2

Decrease the challenge
> Walk out only one step with each hand to lighten the load.
> Wall triceps (p84).

Increase the challenge
> Walk out further.
> Add a third set.

TRAINER TIPS

AVOID LOCKING YOUR ELBOWS AT THE TOP. STOP JUST SHORT OF STRAIGHT.

DON'T LET YOUR BACK SWAY. USE YOUR DEEP ABDOMINALS TO SUPPORT YOUR SPINE.

BE SURE YOU MAINTAIN STRAIGHT, STRONG ALIGNMENT THROUGH YOUR NECK AND UPPER BACK.

STRETCH

SIDE STRETCH AND TRICEP (SEE PAGE 174)

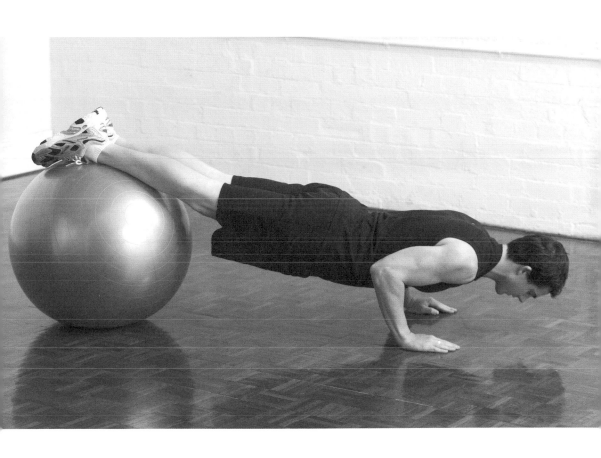

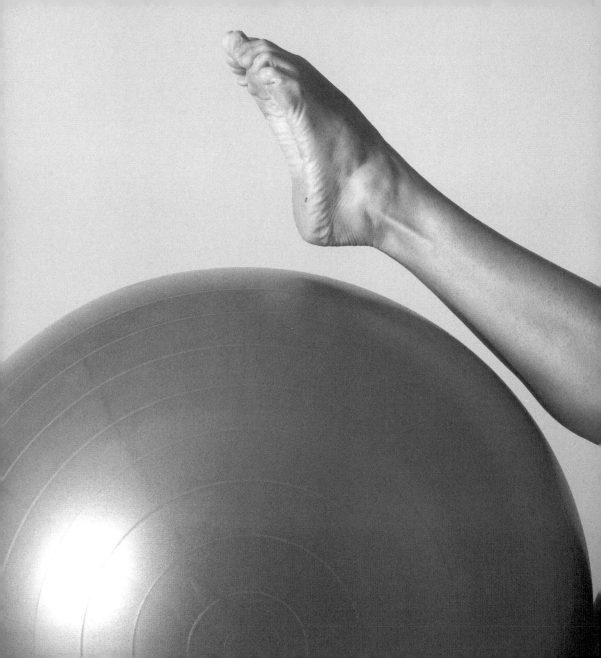

SUPINE ON THE FLOOR

Lying on your back on the floor, with the ball under your legs provides a selection of exercises that range from gentle back health options through to intense strength and stability moves.

All choices combine strength and control. Begin each exercise with your arms resting lightly on the floor beside you. To increase the stability component, raise your forearms off the ground. If you have good control, you are ready to try taking arms off the floor. Working without a wobble while your arms raised is a level of stability to be proud of.

SUPINE BUTTERFLY

precise control

Starting position
> Lie on your back on the floor with your legs together, knees bent and soles of feet resting on the ball.
> Relax your arms by your side.
> Relax your neck and shoulders.

Action
Carefully lower one knee outwards
> Gently draw your lower abdomen towards the floor to activate your core muscles.
> Slowly lower one knee outwards, keeping you back and pelvis still and stable.
> Make sure your other leg stays in position.
> Keep your pelvis level on the floor.
> Do not let your pelvis rotate or your lower back arch.
> Bring the knee back to the midline and repeat with the second leg.

Decrease the challenge
> Perform the movement with your feet on the floor instead of the ball.

Increase the challenge
> Take your foot off the ball and lower your foot to the floor beside the ball.
> Place your arms across your chest.

Go harder
> Raise your arms towards the ceiling. Keep your back flat as you lower the arm, on the same side as the moving leg, sideways towards the floor.

TRAINER TIPS

THIS IS A FINE CONTROL MOVE REQUIRING FOCUS AND AWARENESS.

DO NOT CHEAT BY LETTING THE OTHER KNEE DROP OUTWARD, EVEN A LITTLE.

KEEP YOUR HIPS AND SHOULDERS EVEN AND SQUARE ON THE FLOOR.

STRETCH

ROTATION AND CHEST STRETCH (SEE PAGE 163)

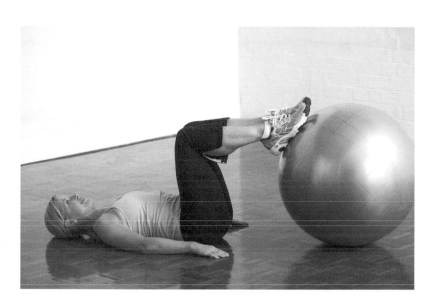

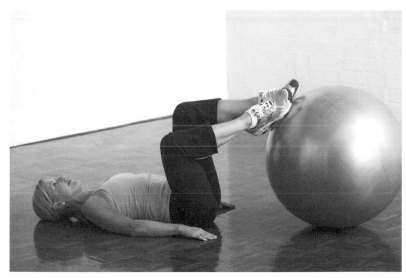

CHEST PRESS WITH BRIDGE AND ROLL

combining chest, back and butt for a total body blitz

Starting position
> Lie with your heels on top of the ball, knees slightly bent.
> Holding your level three weights, place your arms out to the side on the floor level with your shoulders.
> Bend your elbows to 90 degrees so that your hands and forearms are pointing straight up to the ceiling.
> Engage your deep abdominals.

Action
Lift and press
> Push through your heels to raise your hips off the floor.
> Simultaneously perform a chest press, pushing the weights up to meet above your chest.
> Slowly bend your elbows back down and lower your hips in unison.

Decrease the challenge
> Perform arm and leg components individually.

Increase the challenge
> Adding the hamstring roll means more strength and more control.
> Leave your arms on the floor as you lift your hips.
> Perform the chest press as you roll the ball towards you, bending your knees until they are above your hips.

Go harder
> Leave your hips up while you perform 12 x hamstring rolls with chest press, before resting back down.

TRAINER TIPS

KEEP YOUR FEET PULLED BACK SO ONLY THE BACK OF YOUR HEELS ARE IN CONTACT WITH THE BALL.

KEEP YOUR NECK AND SHOULDERS RELAXED.

WHEN ADDING THE HAMSTRING ROLL, THE HARDER YOU PRESS YOUR HEELS DOWN INTO THE BALL, THE MORE YOU WILL WORK YOUR HAMSTRINGS.

STRETCH

ROTATION AND CHEST STRETCH (SEE PAGE 163)

SEATED HAMSTRING STRETCH (SEE PAGE 172)

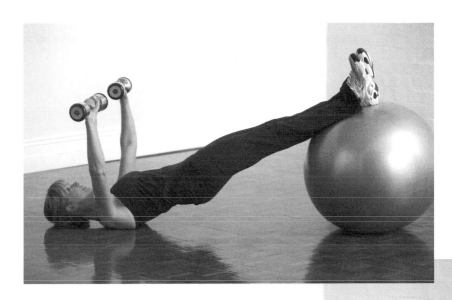

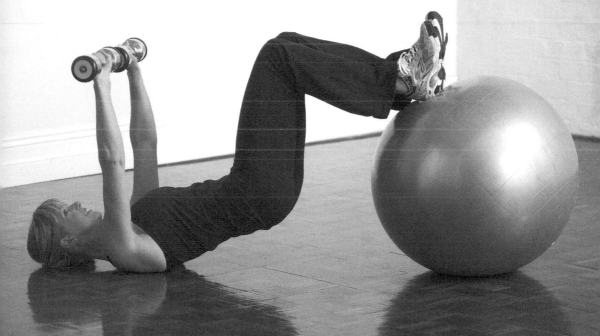

ADDUCTOR LIFT AND ROLL

work your inner thighs like never before

Starting position
> Lie on the floor with your feet around the width of the ball.
> Place the insides of your heels just above the center of the ball, keeping your toes and knees pointing upwards.
> Rest your arms by your side and relax your neck and shoulders.
> Keep your knees slightly bent.

Action
Squeeze, lift and rotate

> Engage your core by drawing your lower abdomen towards the floor.
> Press your heels towards each other to squeeze the ball.
> Keep your knees slightly bent as you raise your hips and pelvis up off the ground.
> Roll the ball sightly to one side then back to the center.
> Lower your hips to the floor ready to repeat the lift and rotate to the second side.
> 10 reps to each side

Decrease the challenge
> Leave out the rotation of the ball. Squeeze the ball and lift your hips, then lower back down x 5.

Increase the challenge
> Raise your hips a little higher.
> Take your arms off the floor and reach them to the ceiling.

TRAINER TIPS

RELAX YOUR NECK AND SHOULDERS.

KEEP YOUR KNEES SLIGHTLY BENT.

MAKE SURE YOU KEEP YOUR KNEES AND TOES POINTING DIRECTLY UPWARDS. NOT INWARDS OR OUTWARDS.

STRETCH

CIRCLE AND HUG (SEE PAGE 162)

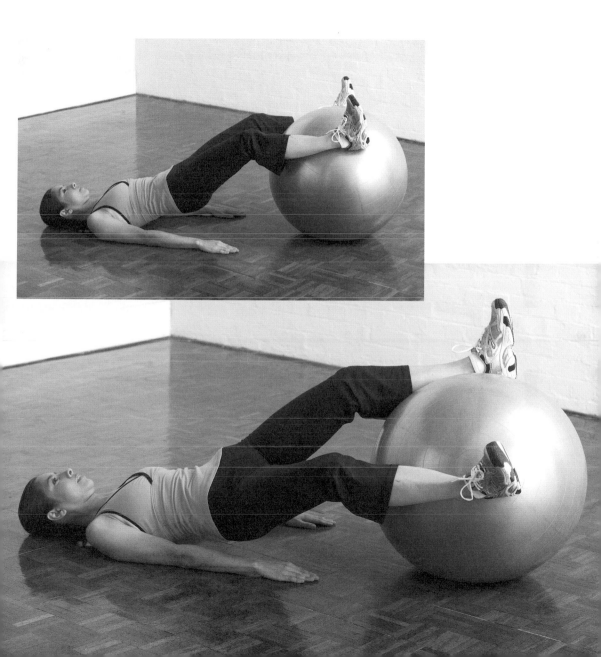

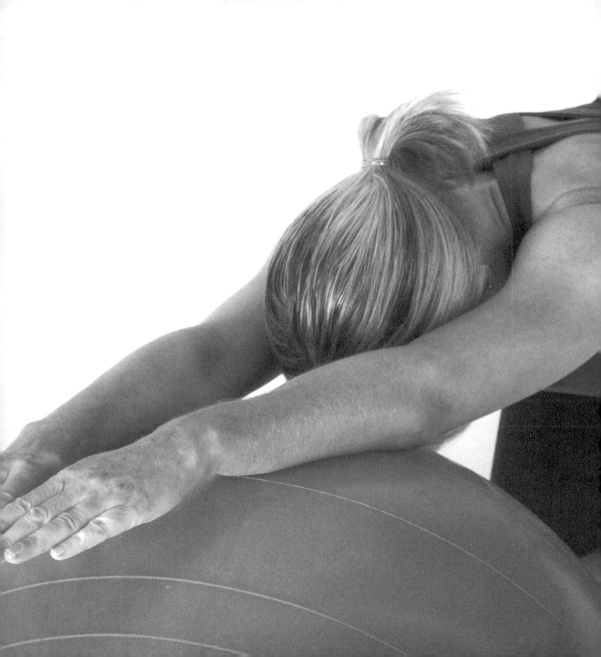

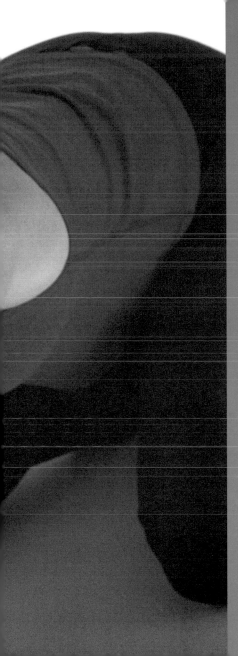

**Stretch for healthy posture
plus free-flowing movement**

Stretching is the most valuable gift you can give your body. Flexibility deserves as much attention and respect as cardio fitness, strengthening, and core work.

It's important to stretch a muscle group after you've worked it. Options to suit each exercise are indicated under trainer tips. To truly balance your life and keep your body moving freely, treat your body and mind to the relax and release program on page 200.

A general stretching regime is the ideal way to keep your body supple and combat common postural problems that can occur as a result of your work or hobbies.

Stretching is most effective when you are warm, such as after you have done other exercise.

Take your stretches to the point of slight stretch only. Do not push to feel discomfort. Hold the stretch without bouncing, while you consciously relax and slow your breath.

Performing a regular flexibilty and mobility program helps to keep you supple, injury-free and moving with ease.

FLEXIBILITY

CIRCLE AND HUG

relax your back

> Lie on your back with your feet on the ball and your hands resting on your knees, which are bent and above your hips.
> Rotate your knees, feet and ball to create slow small circles.
> Slow your breath and focus on relaxing your neck, back and shoulders.
> Repeat for 30 seconds, then hug your knees to your chest.
> Hold the hug for 5 slow breaths before repeating the circles in the other direction.

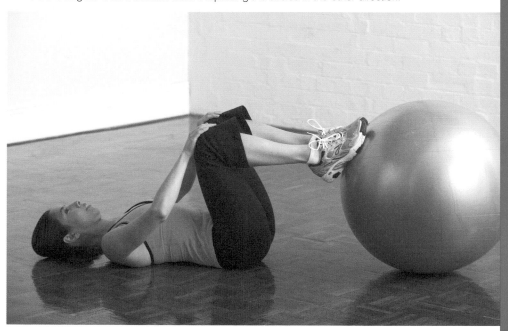

ROTATION AND CHEST STRETCH

iron out the creases in your back while you stretch your pecs

> Lie on your back holding the ball on the floor overhead, knees bent and feet on the floor.
> Slide your fingers down the ball to allow both elbows to rest on the floor level with your shoulders.
> Roll your knees to one side, keeping your opposite elbow on the floor.
> Hold for 10 slow deep breaths allowing your body to ease into the stretch.
> Keep your feet on the floor as you roll over to the second side.

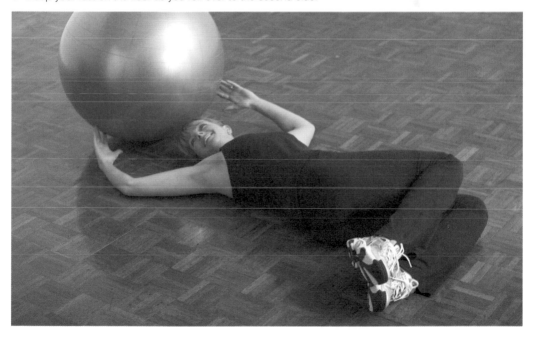

KNEELING
CIRCLES

your back will thank you

> Kneel on the floor. Rest your chest, arms and head on the ball.
> Slowly roll the ball in a circle, allowing your back, pelvis and thighs to follow.
> Relax as you circle slowly 10 times in each direction.

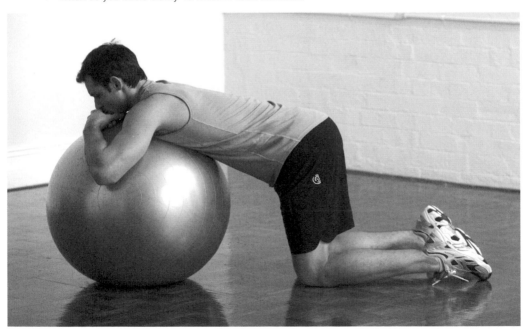

BACK AND
LATS STRETCH

stretch out your back, side and arms

> Kneel upright, your hands resting lightly on the ball in front.
> Sit back over your left heel as you roll the ball forward and to the right.
> Stretch your left arm a little further across feeling the stretch down your side.
> Return to upright kneeling before stretching out the other side.
> Repeat the sequence; rolling from upright kneeling to one side, slowly back up and then over to the other side. Do this 4 times.
> Now hold the outreached position for 10 slow breaths on each side.

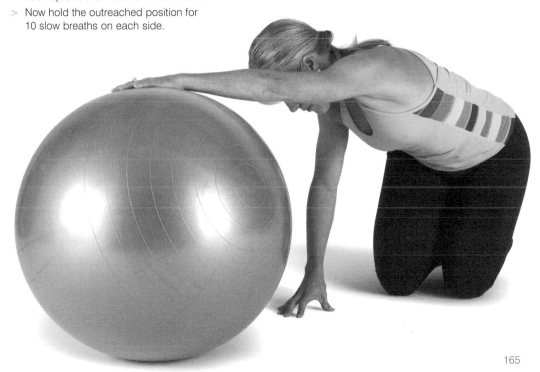

HUG AND ARCH

stretch your spine gently in both directions

> Kneel on the floor, sitting on your heels, toes tucked under.
> Hug the ball and curve your body over it as though molding to the ball.
> Straighten your legs and slowly roll forward.
> Supporting with your hands on the ball, gently lift your chest to arch your back as you roll forward.
> Roll forward and back x 4 then hold the supported arch for 40 to 60 seconds.
> Remember to keep your neck and shoulders relaxed.

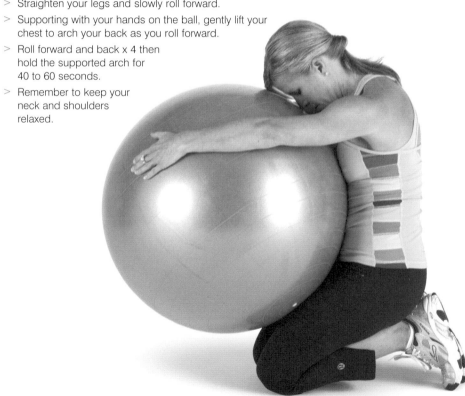

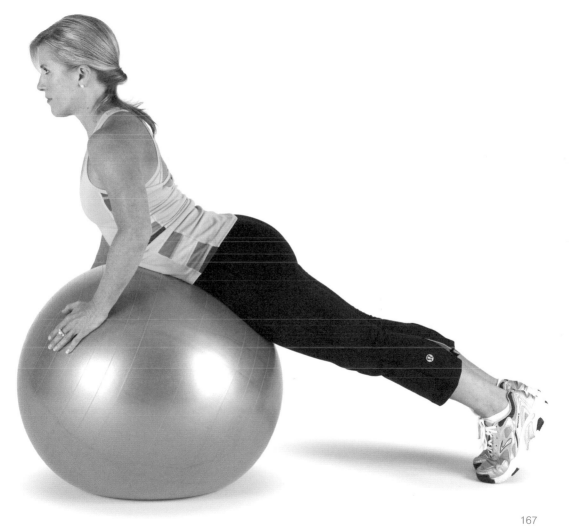

KNEELING SIDE STRETCH

lateral length

> Kneel upright on the floor with your closer hand resting on the ball beside you.

> Roll the ball and your hips away from each other.

> Reach your outside arm up and over to elongate your whole side.

> Breathe while you hold for 40 to 60 seconds each side.

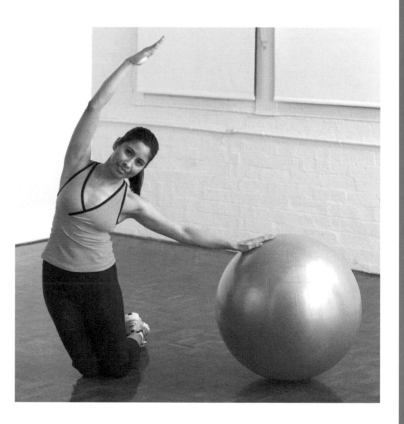

QUADS
STRETCH

stretch out the front of your thigh

> Kneel upright with the ball firmly against your thigh and hip.
> Lie sideways over the ball, sliding your close knee slightly outwards for comfort, with your top arm resting over the ball.
> Lift your outside leg and bend your knee to hold your foot up behind your hip.
> Gently push your foot back into your hand to increase the stretch in your thigh.
> Hold for 10 slow breaths then repeat on the other side.

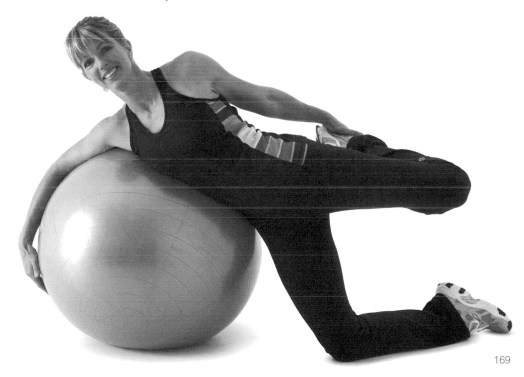

HIP AND
CHEST STRETCH

elongate your hip flexors, pecs and biceps

> Kneel on the floor with your hand resting on the ball to your right.
> Place your left foot well forward in the "marriage proposal" position.
> Lunge forward to open and stretch your right hip.
> Roll the ball back to elongate the front of your right shoulder and arm.
> Hold the position for 40 to 60 seconds then repeat the stretch on the left.

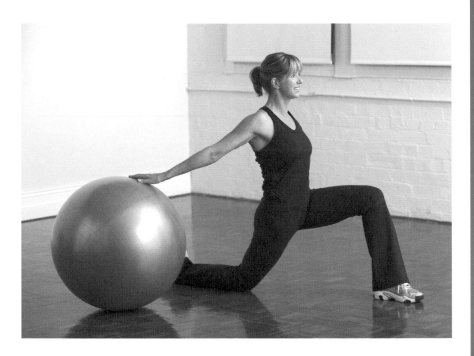

SUPPORTED
CHEST STRETCH

a surprisingly comfortable stretch for your back, abs and chest

> Kneel with your shoelaces flat on the floor.
> Rest the ball on the soles of your shoes behind you.
> Using your hands, low on the ball for support, bend at the hips to touch your tailbone to the ball then gently lower your upper body over the ball.
> Take your hands from behind your back to support your head.
> Gently allow your elbows to open outwards and your head and shoulders to lower back a little more.
> Hold the position for a minute. Replace your hands to the ball, behind your back, bring your chin to your chest and roll back off the ball to upright kneeling.

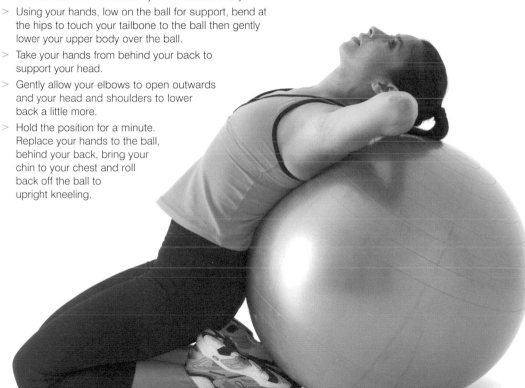

SEATED HAMSTRING STRETCH

stretching out the back of your thighs

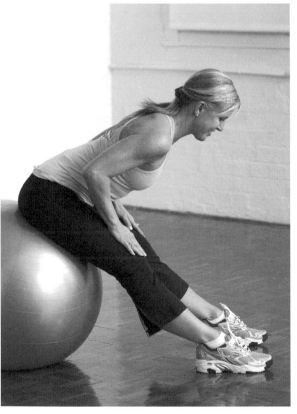

> Sit on the ball with your feet hip width apart and hands resting on your thighs.

> Elongate your spine, lean forward and straighten your knees as you roll the ball backwards.

> Keep your shoulders back and spine long. You should be looking forward at the floor not down at the ball.

> Hold for 10 slow breaths at the point where you feel slight stretch.

POSTERIOR
HIP STRETCH

wobbly but worthwhile

Tightness in the deep muscles
behind the hip is common and
can cause pain or injury. You may
find this stretch wobbly initially,
but practice will allow you to
effectively stretch this potentially
troublesome area.

> Sit slightly forward on your
  ball, with your hands resting
  besides your hips.

> Raise your right foot to cross
  it over your left thigh. Drop the
  right knee outward.

> Lean forward as you roll the
  ball back to feel a stretch
  behind your right hip.

> Hold this stretch for 40 to 60
  seconds before repeating on
  the left.

> If you find it too unstable you
  can try this on a stable chair or
  you can rest one hand on the
  wall beside you as you master
  the ball version.

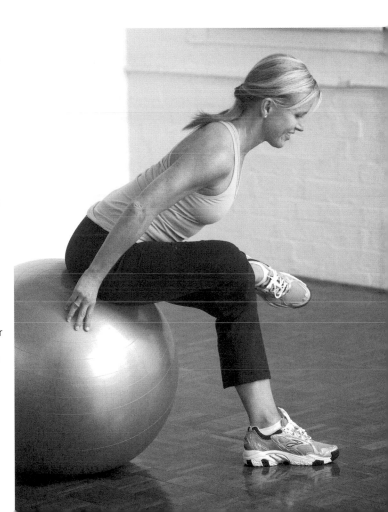

SIDE STRETCH AND TRICEPS

lateral flexibility and triceps length unite

> Sit slightly forward on the ball with your feet and knees wide.

> Bend your right knee and straighten your left as you roll the ball across to that side.

> Reach your right arm up by your ear, bend your elbow to point your forearm to the floor behind your head.

> Use your left hand to gently press downward on the elbow until you feel a slight stretch in the back of your arm.

> Keep your neck long and upright as you hold the stretch for 10 slow breaths.

> Release the stretch and roll to the other side to stretch your left arm.

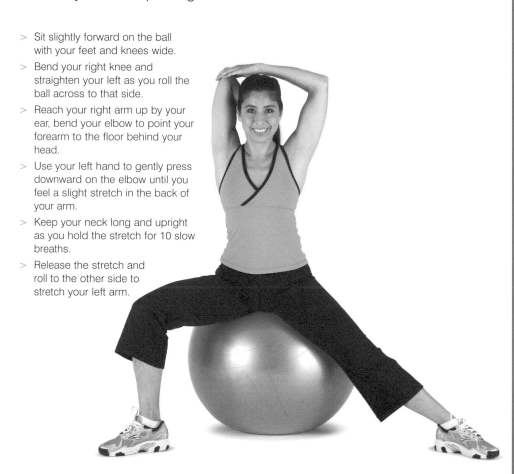

UPPER BACK STRETCH

stretch across your shoulder blades

> Sitting tall on the ball with your feet hip width apart.
> Clasp your hands together and raise them forward to shoulder height.
> Relax your shoulders downwards and gently push your palms forward to round your upper back and stretch across your shoulder blades, hold for 5 slow breaths.
> Now reach your clasped palms up over head, release them at the top and allow them to float back down by your sides.
> Repeat x 3

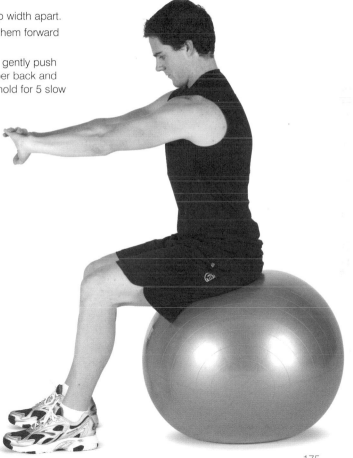

SEATED ROTATION

keep your spine mobile

> Sit tall on the ball with your feet hip width apart or closer.
> Turn your upper body to the left.
> Reach your right arm across your body, placing the hand on the outside of your left thigh.
> Sit tall and turn as far as you can comfortably, as though looking behind.
> Hold the position for 5 slow breaths, repeat to each side x 2.

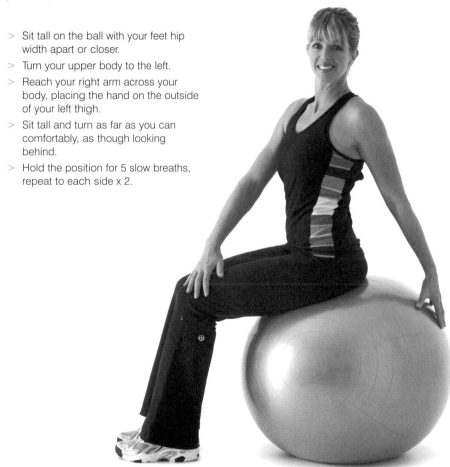

NECK
SEMI-CIRCLES

go gently with your neck

Move your neck only within comfort and take care to keep the movement slow and smooth

> Sit tall on the ball, with your arms relaxed by your sides
> Turn your neck to look over one shoulder
> Draw a semi-circle. Glide your chin slowly downwards, across your chest and back up to look over the other shoulder.
> Slowly x 2 each direction.

Lateral stretch

> Now, looking straight ahead, tilt your head to one side taking your ear towards your shoulder.
> Keep the opposite arm down.
> Hold for 3 relaxed breaths.
> Roll your shoulders, up, back and down x 3 before repeating to the second side.

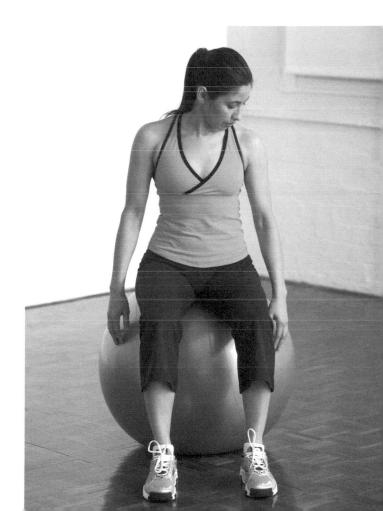

WALL STRETCH

a wonderful way to stretch head to toe

> Stand with your ball at the wall at chest height.
> Walk forward to roll the ball up the wall until your arms are reaching high above you.
> Step in under the ball to feel the stretch through your arms, lats and abdominals.
> Hold x 5 slow breaths, roll back down and repeat x 3.

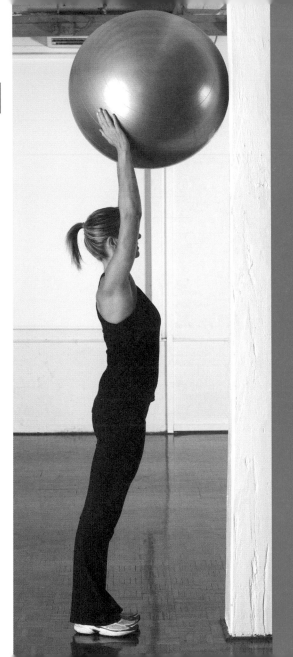

STANDING HIP FLEXOR STRETCH

this stretch requires balance and control

A fabulous way to elongate and open the whole front of your body and stretch your chest, abdominals and hip flexors.

> Stand and roll the ball back behind you catching it with your toes.
> The ball must be rolled back sufficiently, so that it is resting under your foot only and your raised knee is extended back behind you.
> Bend your front leg as you roll the ball backwards to gently stretch your hip.
> Remain upright through your torso.
> Raise your arms in front to chest height.
> Turn your palms up and your thumbs outwards and glide your arms out to be level with your shoulders to open and stretch across your chest.
> Hold for 10 slow breaths on each leg.

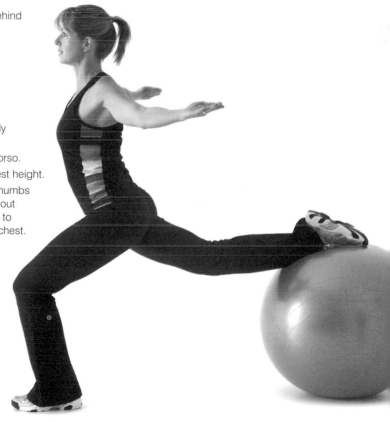

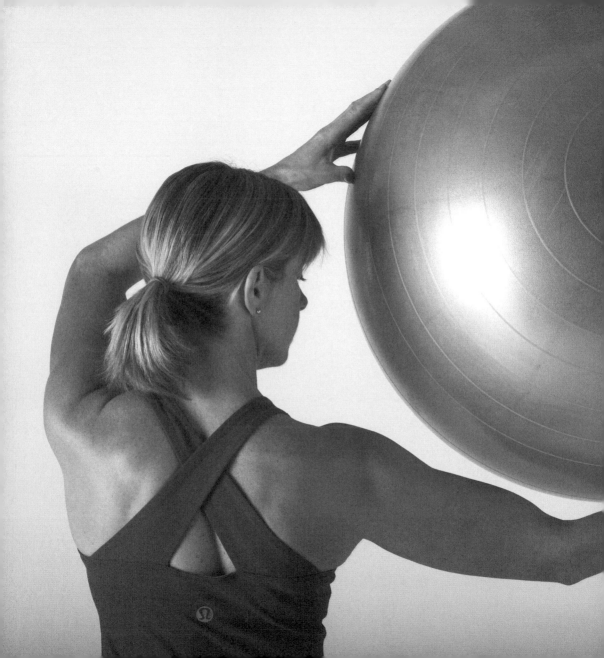

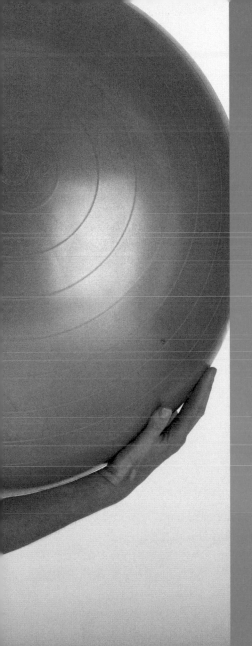

The exercises in *Get on the Ball for Great Abs* can be combined in an unlimited number of ways. You can performa a section of exercises to suit your aims and abilities. Alternatively, you can explore these physiotherapy-designed programs, which have been created to help you meet your goals and match your needs. The programs range from gentle to tough levels of difficulty.

Need a short workout? If you are looking for the 10-minute morning wake up or evening unwind, or you suffer the consequences of sitting at a computer all day the 10-minute quick-fix programs are for you.

Vary your training and be sure to balance your strength work with the flexibility. Your body will thank you.

Enjoy the programs and reap the results of fitter, toned abs and a strong stable body.

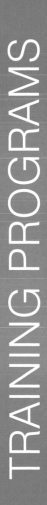

TRAINING PROGRAMS

GETTING STARTED

gentle mobility, stability and familiarity

Ease into user-friendly ball exercises to help you get moving,
find your core, and develop confidence on the ball.

1
Shoulder rolls
page 36

2
Climb the Ladder
page 37

3
Pelvic Clock
page 38

4
Upper Back
Warm-up
page 39

5
Side Tap
page 54

6
Wall Hover
page 82

7
Seated
Semi-squat
page 88

8
Bands and Biceps
(light resistance only)
page 90

9
Breaststroke (just
one arm at a time)
page 130

10
Supine Butterfly
page 154

11
Circle and Hug
page 162

12
Kneeling Circles
page 164

13
Seated Rotation
page 176

CARDIO BLITZ

bounce into action

Get your ball and body bouncing with an upbeat, low impact cardio session. Use this as a warm up, a fun bouncy workout or combine it with your favorite strength program for a great mix of cardio, strength, and core.

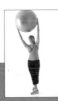

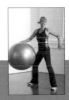

1
Rolling Side to Side, Arm Circles
page 40

2
Reach and Sit
page 46

3
Step and Bounce
page 58

4
Curl Swing
page 59

5
Rainbow
page 61

6
Boxer Bounce
page 62

7
Skip and Bounce
page 63

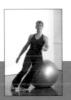
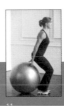

8
Heels Forward
page 67

9
Star Jumps
page 68

10
Ski Jumps
page 69

11
Seated Semi-squat
page 88

12
Back and Lats stretch
page 165

13
Hug and Arch
page 166

14
Quads Stretch
page 169

TOTAL WORKOUT 1

get going

Get your fitness regime started using straightforward exercises on the ball.
Be sure to stretch after each exercise.

1
Circle and Reach
page 45

2
Step and Bounce
page 58

3
Curl and Swing
page 59

4
Reach and Sit
page 46

5
Reach Across
page 41

6
Ball-assisted
Lunge
page 72

7
Wall Triceps
page 84

8
Bands and Biceps
page 90

9
Lateral Arm Raise
page 92

10
Knee Roll
page 108

11
Side Lean
and Raise
page 126

12
Breaststroke
page 130

13
Scissors
page 138

14
Prone Walk Out
page 146

TOTAL WORKOUT 2

a strong workout inside and out, head to toe

Step up your workout, mixing cardio and strength.
Follow each exercise with the relevant stretch.

1
Circle and Reach
page 45

2
Standing Back
Roll
page 48

3
Reach Across
page 41

4
Basic Bounce
page 66

5
Heels Forward
page 67

6
Wall Walk
page 80

7
Lat Pull Down
page 96

8
Climb the Rope
page 104

9
Roll Away V
page 110

10
Supine Glide
page 120

11
Leg Raise Forward
and Back
page 124

12
Prone Row
with Band
page 134

13
Crossed Leg
Extension
page 140

14
Chest Press with
Bridge and Roll
page 156

TOTAL WORKOUT 3

a total body challenge

A bouncy warm-up followed by a longer tougher program to further challenge strength and control.

1
Rolling Arm
Circles
page 40

2
Rolling Reach
Across
page 41

3
Double Step
and Bounce
page 60

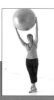

4
Rainbow
page 61

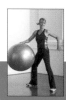

5
Boxer Bounce
page 62

6
Star Jumps
page 68

7
Ski Jumps
page 69

8
Single Leg Lunge
page 74

9
Triceps with Band
page 94

10
Lateral Arm Raise
page 92

11
Curl and Reach
page 100

12
Curl and Extend
page 101

13
Lat Pull Down
page 96

14
Ball Hover
page 112

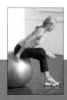

15
Supine Rotation
page 116

16
Supine Pec Pass
page 118

17
Leg Raise
Forward and Back
page 124

18
Breast Stroke
page 130

19
Prone Row
page 134

20
Diamond Leg Lift
page 142

21
Uneven Push-up
page 148

22
Triceps Push-up
page 150

23
Chest Press with
Bridge and Roll
page 156

24
Adductor Lift
and Roll
page 158

25
Rotation and Chest
Stretch
page 163

26
Posterior Hip
Stretch
page 173

27
Standing Hip and
Flexor Stretch
page 179

POST-PREGNANCY

safe effective exercise to help you get back in shape after baby

Get on the ball to optimize your health and fitness during this time after baby.
Consult with your physical therapist before commencing exercise. Perform a
slow pelvic floor lift after every third exercise.

1
Shoulder Rolls
page 36

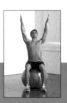

2
Arm Circles
page 36

3
Pelvic Clock
page 38

4
Upper Back
Warm-up
page 39

5
Side Tap
page 54

6
Rotate and Control
(Optional Leg Lift)
page 176

7
Seated Semi-
squat
page 88

8
Wall Triceps
page 84

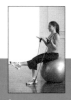

9
Bands and Biceps
page 90

10
Lateral Arm Raise
page 92

11
Kneeling Circles
page 164

12
Seated Hamstring Stretch (Sit with
legs a little wider than hip width.)
page 172

BACK IN ACTION

Back health on the ball

Keep your back healthy with sensible, safe exercises to strengthen and stabilize your spine.
If you have an existing back problem consult with your physical therapist before commencing
any exercise, and listen to your body. Discontinue any move that causes discomfort.

1
Shoulder rolls
page 36

2
Upper Back
warm-up
page 39

3
Pelvic Clock
page 38

4
Seated Walk
page 52

5
Side Step
page 53

6
Side Tap
page 54

7
Seated Rotation
page 176

8
Wall Walk
page 80

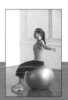

9
Wall Hover
page 82

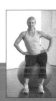

10
Breaststroke
page 130

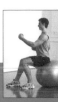

11
Kneeling
Extension
page 132

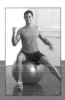

12
Prone Row (no
band or weights)
page 134

13
Supine Butterfly
page 154

14
Seated Rotation
page 176

RELEASE YOUR BACK

ease away the tension

Perform these mobility and flexibility moves on the ball slowly
to free your back of tension and tightness.

1
Neck Semi-circles
page 177

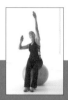

2
Climb the Ladder
page 37

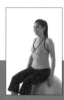

3
Shoulder Rolls
page 36

4
Arm Circles
page 36

5
Reach Across
page 41

6
Kneeling Back
and Shoulder Roll
page 42

7
Kneeling Circles
page 164

8
Back and
Lats stretch
page 165

9
Hug and Arch
page 166

10
Hip and
Chest Stretch
page 170

11
Side Stretch
and Triceps
page 174

12
Seated Hamstring
Stretch
page 172

13
Seated Rotation
page 176

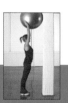

14
Wall Stretch
page 178

ABS AND BACK

a toned torso, front and back

A tough workout front and back. Everyone wants strong abs.
Giving equal attention to abs and back makes for a strong midsection
and fabulous posture. Remember to stretch after each exercise.

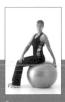

1
Standing
Back Roll
page 48

2
Seated Rotation
page 176

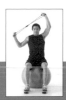

3
Lat Pull Down
page 96

4
Curl and Reach
page 100

5
Curl and Step
page 102

6
Curl and
Side reach
page 103

7
Supine Glide
page 120

8
Ball Hover
page 112

9
Breaststroke
page 130

10
Prone Row
with Band
page 134

11
Scissors
page 138

12
Back and
Lats Stretch
page 165

13
Supported
Chest Stretch
page 171

14
Hug and Arch
page 166

ARMS, CHEST AND UPPER BACK

upper body conditioning for form and function

Use this program to strengthen your upper body.

1
Boxer Bounce
page 62

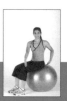

2
Waist Warm-up
page 39

3
Reach Across
page 41

4
Bands and Biceps
page 90

5
Lateral Arm Raise
page 92

6
Lat Pull Down
page 96

7
Supine Pec Pass
page 118

8
Prone Row
with Band
page 134

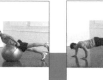

9
Prone Triceps
with Band
page 136

10
Uneven Push-up
page 148

11
Chest Press with
Bridge and Roll
page 156

12
Supported
Chest Stretch
page 171

13
Back and
Lats stretch
page 165

14
Hug and Arch
page 166

THIGHS AND BUTT

a below the belt blitz

Hone in on your thighs and gluteals for a leg and bottom workout you will really feel.

1
Reach and Sit
page 46

2
Curl and Swing
page 59

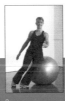

3
Ski Jumps
page 69

4
Lean and Lift
page 76

5
Seated Semi-squat
page 88

6
Leg Raise Forward and Back
page 124

7
Scissors
page 138

8
Crossed Leg Extension
page 140

9
Diamond Leg Lift
page 142

10
Adductor Lift and Roll
page 158

11
Hug and Arch
page 166

12
Quads Stretch
page 169

13
Seated Hamstring Stretch
page 172

14
Posterior Hip Stretch
page 173

CORE CONTROL

building sound foundations

Work on your core stability for great balance.

1
Shoulder Rolls
page 36

2
Waist Warm-up
page 38

3
Pelvic Clock
page 38

4
Seated Walk
page 52

5
Side Step
page 53

6
Rotate and Control
with Leg Lift
page 176

7
Wall Walk
page 80

8
Wall Hover
page 82

9
Prone Walk-out
page 146

10
Overhead Control
page 106

11
Side Lean
and Raise
page 126

12
Supine Butterfly
page 154

13
Rotation and
Chest Stretch
page 163

14
Seated Rotation
page 176

STRONG AND STABLE

working inside and out

Mixing strength and stability will have you standing tall proud, strong, and injury-free.

1
Circle and Reach
page 45

2
Boxer Bounce
page 62

3
Single Leg Lunge
with Tricep Row
page 75

4
Lean and Lift
page 76

5
Lat Pull Down
page 96

6
Curl and Reach
page 100

7
Roll Away V
page 110

8
Supine Pec Pass
page 118

9
Side Lean
and Leg Lift
page 126

10
Uneven Push-up
page 150

11
Scissors
page 138

12
Adductor Lift
and Roll
page 158

13
Back and
Lats Stretch
page 165

14
Hip and
Chest Stretch
page 170

CORE STRENGTH CHALLENGE

a true test of control for those with experience

Test your stability and strength with this advanced combination of strength and stability options.

1
Reach and Sit
page 46

2
Skip and Bounce
page 63

3
Single Leg Lunge
page 74

4
Lateral Arm Raise
(Single Arm Leg Up)
page 93

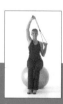

5
Lat Pull Down
(Single Arm and Leg)
page 94

6
Curl and Reach (Add
Opposite Leg Extend)
page 100

7
Ball Hover
(Add Leg Lift)
page 112

8
Leg Raise (Hold
Leg Up and Circle)
page 124

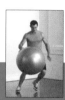

9
Diamond Leg Lift
page 142

10
Triceps Push-up
page 150

11
Chest Press with
Bridge and Roll
page 156

12
Adductor Lift and
Roll (Arms Up)
page 158

13
Wall Stretch
page 178

14
Standing Hip and
Flexor Stretch
page 179

MORNING WAKE-UP CALL

kick start your day

Get the most out of your morning workout.

1
Shoulder Rolls
page 36

2
Neck Semi-circles
page 177

3
Climb the Ladder
page 37

4
Waist Warm-Up
page 38

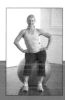
5
Pelvic Clock
page 38

6
Upper Back
Warm-up
page 39

7
Circle and Reach
page 45

8
Standing
Back Roll
page 48

9
Ball-assisted
Lunge
page 72

10
Wall Stretch
page 178

EVENING UNWIND

roll away the tension

Stretch, relax and breathe to blow away the tension of the day.

1
Roll Side to Side
shoulder rolls
page 40

2
Rolling side to
side Arm circles
page 40

3
Kneeling Back
and Shoulder Roll
page 42

4
Back and
Lats stretch
page 165

5
Kneeling Circles
page 164

6
Hug and Arch
page 166

7
Hip and
Chest Stretch
page 170

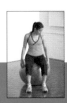

8
Seated Hamstring
Stretch
page 172

9
Upper Back
Stretch
page 175

10
Seated Rotation
page 176

11
Neck Semi-circles
page 177

12
Wall Stretch
page 178

COMPUTER QUICK-FIX

combat the slouches and tightness that go with the job.

Sitting at the computer or steering wheel compromises posture and leads to muscle weakness and tightness. Counteract this with a few simple exercises to stretch out the tightness and strengthen those areas that feel weak.

1
Shoulder Rolls
page 36

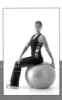

2
Seated Rotation
page 176

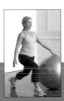

3
Ball-assisted
Lunge
page 73

4
Kneeling
Extension
page 132

5
Prone Row
with Band
page 134

6
Crossed Leg
Extension
page 140

7
Hug and Arch
page 166

8
Hip and
Chest Stretch
page 170

9
Supported
Chest Stretch
page 171

10
Neck Semi-circles
page 177

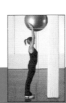

11
Wall Stretch
page 178

RELAX AND RELEASE

because you deserve it

Add relaxing music and slow, even breathing to these moves to stretch, relax, and release. Start lying on the floor, with your legs resting on the ball. Take a few minutes to slow down your breathing and relax.

1
Circle and Hug
page 162

2
Rotation and
Chest Stretch
page 163

3
Kneeling Circles
page 164

4
Back and
Lats Stretch
page 165

5
Hug and Arch
page 166

6
Kneeling
Side Stretch
page 168

7
Quads Stretch
page 169

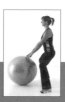

8
Seated Hamstring
Stretch
page 172

9
Shoulder Rolls
page 36

10
Neck Semi-circles
page 177

11
Standing Back
Roll
page 48

12
Circle and Reach
page 45

ABOUT THE AUTHOR

Lisa Westlake is a physiotherapist, mother of two and highly regarded Australian fitness instructor and presenter. Her first book, *Strong to the Core*, has sold over 100,000 copies. Lisa was awarded Australian Fitness Professional of the Year in 2000 and Australian Fitness Presenter of the Year in 2003.

She left her full-time physiotherapy position in road trauma intensive care in 1995 to create her business "Physical Best", which develops and provides quality exercise programs for people of all abilities and needs. Lisa is known as the pioneer of fitball training in Australia, and in addition to *Strong to the Core*, she has also produced six fitness DVDs.

Lisa is a highly regarded national and international presenter, lectures in several universities, writes for fitness magazines, and has a popular health and fitness talkback segment on Melbourne's ABC Saturday Morning Radio.

ACKNOWLEDGEMENTS

Writing a book is a little like composing a symphony. It's one thing to create the music but it takes a range of instruments and musicians to perform it in perfect harmony. There are many in my orchestra to acknowledge.

Thanks to Stuart Neal and ABC Books for giving me the opportunity to write again and to the international publishers who have taken my exercises to people far away.

A standing ovation for Jody Lee, my conductor, who so cheerfully and patiently brought the symphony together with true editorial style.

To my fellow musicians for their patience and wonderful work in front of the camera: Liz Dene; Yani Burmeister; Sean Logue; and Jeannette Lefrandt, not only for her fabulous photogenic form but also for her unrelenting 24- hour support and friendship.

My appreciation to the people backstage: Ingo Voss for his fabulous flair for design; Julieann Howard for her skill and creativity behind the lens; Danielle Shukur for her make-up and styling; and Marc at CI Studios for making the studio shoot a dream.

For equipment and clothing, my thanks go to lululemon athletica in Melbourne for their generous supply of fabulous fitness wear, Brooks shoes for making sure our feet looked equally great, to Fitball Therapy and Training, The Australian Barbell company and QPEC Fitness Solutions for the balls, hand weights and resistance bands respectively.

To friends, colleagues and class participants, thank you for your encouragement and inspiration.

A big thank you to John Davies who has always been there for me, with business advice, encouragement, support and a small kick up the — when I need one! Thanks go to Sue Williams, a special friend and a fabulous manager. Thanks too to Belinda and Megan who were so helpful in the busiest time of writing and especially to Margaret Lindholm for her willingness to 'step in' when I needed to "step out".

Most importantly, to my front row audience, who give me feedback on all my works in progress and cheer me on regardless: Dave, Daniel and Jessica. Thank you just for being you.

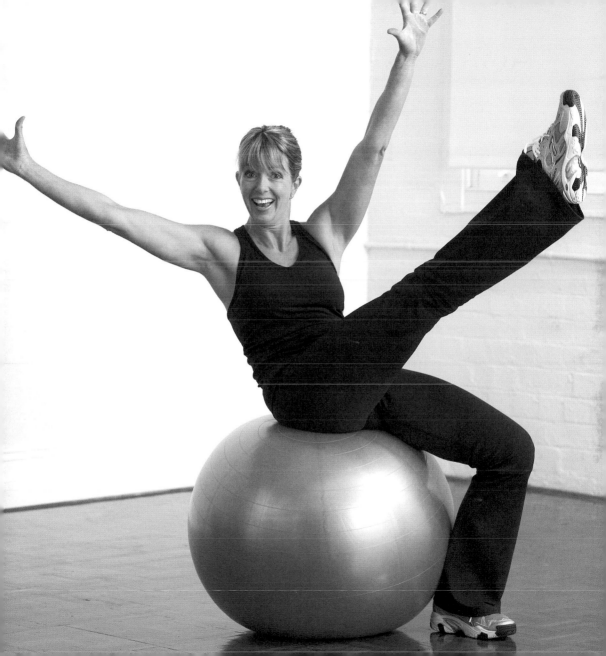